Shadows of Mawangdui

Animating the Silk *Daoyintu*

Ronald C. Smith
&
Antonio M. Carmone

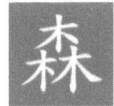

Three Pines Press
St. Petersburg, FL 33713
www.threepinespress.com

© 2022 by Ronald C. Smith and Antonio M. Carmone

All rights reserved. No part of this book may be reproduced in any form or by any means, electronic or mechanical, including photocopying, recording, or by any information storage and retrieval system, without permission in writing from the publisher.

9 8 7 6 5 4 3 2 1

Printed in the United States of America
This edition is printed on acid-free paper that meets the American National Standard Institute Z39. 48 Standard.
Distributed in the United States by Three Pines Press.

Cover Art: *Daoyintu* image, refined by Victoria R. Smith.
Cover Design: Brent Christopher Wulf

Library of Congress Cataloging-in-Publication Data
Names: Smith, Ronald C., 1946- author. | Carmone, Antonio M., 1940- author.
Title: Shadows of Mawangdui : animating the silk daoyintu / Ronald C. Smith & Antonio M. Carmone.
Description: St. Petersburg, FL : Three Pines Press, 2022. | Includes bibliographical references and index.
Identifiers: LCCN 2022021351 | ISBN 9781931483704 (paperback)
Subjects: LCSH: Huang Lao bo shu. | Dao yin. | Exercise--Religious aspects--Taoism. | Healing--Religious aspects--Taoism. | Medicine, Chinese
Classification: LCC RA781.85 .S65 2022 | DDC 299.5/14--dc23/eng/20220603
LC record available at https://lccn.loc.gov/2022021351

Contents

Acknowledgments	vii
Introduction	1
1. An Enigma at *Mawangdui*	4
2. *Daoyintu* Connections	12
3. Practice Guidelines	18
4. Movements 1 through 11	25
5. Movements 12 through 22	49
6. Movements 23 through 33	73
7. Movements 34 through 44	97
8. Interpretations and Combinations	120
9. Self and Self-Care	130
10. Initiating Engagement	135
11. Your *Daoyintu* Experience	141
Appendices	144
Bibliography	149
The Authors	153
Index	157

List of Illustrations

Fig. 1: Original Mawangdui silk drawing. L0040263 *Daoyintu*—Chart for leading and guiding people in exercise. Credit: Wellcome Collection, London. images@wellcome.ac.uk http://wellcomeimages.org Daoyin tu

Fig. 2: Reconstructed image of the *Daoyintu*. Souce: same as Fig. 1, L0036007 Poster 20th Century Published: Copyrighted work available under Creative Commons Attribution only license CC BY 4.0 http://creativecom-mons.org/licenses/by/4.0/

Fig. 3 Medical texts attached to the *Daoyintu*, used with permission of Dolly Yang.

Fig. 4: The top row of *Daoyintu*

Fig. 5: The second row of *Daoyintu*

Fig. 6: The third row of *Daoyintu*

Fig. 7: The bottom row of *Daoyintu*

Fig. 8: *Daoyintu* #24

Fig. 9: *Daoyintu* #41

Fig. 10: *Daoyintu* #38

Fig. 11: Modified *Daoyintu* #38

Fig. 12: *Daoyintu* #42

Fig. 13: *Daoyintu* #9 and 14

Fig. 14: *Daoyintu* #2, 8, 36, 12

Fig. 15: *Daoyintu* #20, 15, 35

Fig. 16: *Daoyintu* #24, 8, 1, 43

Fig. 17: *Daoyintu* #25, 27, 42, 18

Fig. 18: *Daoyintu* #38, 19

Fig. 19: *Daoyintu* #12

Fig. 20: *Daoyintu* #24

Fig. 21: Modified *Daoyintu* #38

Acknowledgments

This book has taken a long time to evolve. It began in the late 1990s with our studies of taiji quan and various energy practices with Master Li Changduo and Madam Hu Yang in Leuven, Belgium. In 2002, Madam Hu Yang told our class that we were going to learn some new exercises. These new exercises turned out to be the *Daoyintu*, which were depicted on a silk manuscript found at the Mawangdui tombs sealed more than 2000 years ago. Madam Hu Yang never explained where she learned the movements, but she freely passed them on to us. Each student received a copy of the *Daoyintu* figures, which can be seen in Chapter One, Figure 2. As she taught each movement, one of the authors kept detailed notes and stick-figure drawings in order to reconstruct the movements in case memory failed. Her interpretations of the forty-four *Daoyintu* figures are the basis for the movements presented in this book, augmented by twenty years of the authors experience practicing, teaching, and refining them.

By 2006 we had taken separate paths both as learners and teachers. Tony received an Acupuncture Degree from the University of Portsmouth, UK, and Ron, who had moved to Texas, studied various bodywork therapies and taught thousands of taiji quan classes. Being friends, we stayed in touch, but it really wasn't until 2016, when we met at Tony's house in Florida, and practiced all forty-four *Daoyintu* movements, that we fully realized there had been hidden treasure in Hu Yang's lessons. In May 2020, Tony suggested that the two of us collaborate on a book.

Referring to the hand-written instruction book, we re-tried each movement on our own, attempting to reimagine the ancient wisdom that created them. We drew on lessons from past teachers and continued to learn with our students. With plenty of time on our hands and Skype sessions twice a week the book started to take form. This creative process, along with our academic research, gave us new insights into the possible meaning of the *Daoyintu* images, as well as about energy flow.

To augment our understanding of the *Daoyintu*, we referred to experts who have written well-researched books in English dealing with this subject. Among them are Donald Harper, whose book *Early Chinese Medical Literature: The Mawangdui Medical Manuscripts* is seminal. He initially studied reproductions of the original material in 1977 and later, in consultation with a group of Chinese researchers, he had access to the original material. As such he is a main source of Chinese translation and interpretation.

Other key academic sources are Livia Kohn's book *Chinese Healing Exercises: The Tradition of Daoyin* and her edited volume, *Daoist Meditation and Longevity Techniques*. A particularly insightful piece in the latter is "Gymnastics: The Ancient Tradition" by Catherine Despeux. We have also appreciated the perspective of Vivienne Lo's translation of the *Yinshu*, a contemporaneous health manuscript. *Creativity and Daoism*, by Chung-yuan Chang, was also a very helpful source. Their knowledge of ancient Chinese culture, Daoism, and the Chinese language have helped us understand what may have been intended by the creator(s) of these movements.

We want to thank Madam Hu Yang, who taught us the *Daoyintu* and set us on the path to this book. Additionally, we are sincerely grateful to a number of teachers, whose in-person and written instruction over the years helped us understand the physical and energetic aspects of the *Daoyintu*. They include Master Li Changduo, Master Kai-Han Lo, Madame Gei-Lin Liu, and Master Freddie Van Hove, from Brussels; Master Su Yuchang in Taiwan; Master Simon Lau at Eastern Horizons Studio in London, Master Leng Tang in Florida, Master Lam Kam Chuen, Dr. Stephen T. Chang, Mimi Kuo-Deemer, and Wong Kiew Kit. Our dedicated students Jim Fesler, Diana Casabar, Kathy Tipps, Tom Gartside, Dr. Chikita Maus, Hector Petroni, and Steve Russell helped us refine movements and validate their effects.

This book would not have existed without the superb efforts of the publisher and chief editor of Three Pines Press, Thomas L. Moscarillo and Livia Kohn, who have been an absolute pleasure to work with throughout the entire process. Thanks, also, to Dr. Dolly Yang for reviewing our manuscript, providing insights and advice for improvement and for generously making her doctoral thesis on "Prescribing Guiding and Pulling," available to us.

Finally, we thank our families, who provided inspiration and support over the years. Our wives, Wanda Smith and JoEllen Carmone, were great encouragers, sounding-boards, and reviewers of our writing efforts. Ron's daughter, Victoria, contributed artwork, photographed the movements, edited the photos and provided French translation.

Note to the Reader: The authors and the publisher specifically disclaim liability for any loss or risk incurred by the use or application of any of the contents of this book.

Introduction

The *Daoyintu* is one of the earliest documents on Chinese health and energy cultivation practice. As Yu Gongbao notes,

> Its oldest and most diverse form is *daoyin*, which holds an important position in the traditional Chinese art of preserving one's health. *Dao* refers to the fact that physical movements are guided by the strength of the mind and in turn stimulate the internal flow of *qi* within the body. *Yin* means that with the aid of physical movements, *qi* can reach the bodily extremities (e.g., the fingers, feet, and head). (1995, 8)

The term *daoyin* consists of two characters, that each have ten meanings. To begin, *dao* 導 means "to guide." It is different from the character for *dao* or "way" 道, the root of the word Daoism. To avoid confusion of English usages, we will use the term Daoism when referring to the philosophy and religion. Also, note that the Chinese character for *yin* 陰, as in yin and yang is different from the Chinese character for *yin* 引 in *daoyin*, which means "to pull" or "stretch." *Tu* 圖, finally, means "map" and can be interpreted as "chart."

After many years of learning, practicing and teaching, we have observed that no one practices exactly the same form of *daoyin*, qigong, or taiji quan. So, there are in a sense as many different forms of energy cultivation as the number of people who practice them. The way each person performs a *daoyin*, qigong or taiji quan form is a variation on the same theme of moving and guiding *qi* for greater energy, health and healing. We have avoided using the term qigong, because its meaning has become so diverse. Instead, we use the term *daoyin* for the energy practice and *Daoyintu* for the original drawings of the forty-four figures that form the basis of our book.

Because the *Daoyintu* manuscript was damaged, the postures, their names, and their purpose are only partially understood. The incomplete static figures are akin to shadows that may be interpreted in many ways.

We offer movements that tap into ancient wisdom which have both specific and general application to various health and energy conditions. When you have learned the physical movements, you can explore them in energetic depth. We provide some techniques to gain insight for a self-care plan. Then, if you wish, you can delve deeper into more esoteric practices of ritual and meditation. We have found these play important roles when doing *daoyin*.

Doing these movements can give you feelings of release and a profound sense of connection. Both authors have had spiritual experiences while practicing the animal movements of the *Daoyintu* and the *Wuqinxi* (Five Animals' Frolics), through the direct and indirect teachings of Master Simon Lau who teaches at the Eastern Horizon Studios in South Kensington, London.

Over time, everyone builds up a set of personal healing actions, that can range from simply rubbing a sore area to doing a complex stretch, energy form, acupressure, acupuncture, or dietary practice. We hope you will take the portions of this book that appeal to you and add them to your complementary health practice, making informed decisions and taking responsibility for your own self-care. You can, and should, go further to re-imagine and re-create new sets of movements and practices inspired by the *Daoyintu* into your own personal repertoire.

We do not feel that we should make any promises about results from doing the activities in this book. We have our own personal results, but your results may vary. We hope you enjoy doing them as much as we and our students do, but relax, and do not try too hard.

Boundless Possibilities

Penetrating Yin and Yang,
Inside the Abdomen,
Pulling the Warm Ailment,
Looking Up and Shouting,
Crane Calling,
Monkey Bawling,
Gibbon Jumping,
Bear Rambling,
Dragon Ascending.
The Uncarved Block Awaits.

Chapter One

An Enigma at Mawangdui

An Ancient Library for Health

It's the time of the Han dynasty, which lasted from 206 BCE to 220 CE, Chancellor Li Cang, also known as the Marquis of Dai and his wife, Xin Zhui, are preparing to bury their son in the family tomb at Mawangdui near Changsha in Hunan. In the beliefs of that time, the "soul" was split at death and part of it remained on earth, associated with the body of the deceased. This essence of their son, judged to be in his thirties, could still learn and develop skills for the afterlife. Thus, a considerable library was interred with him. As Livia Kohn notes,

> In Han understanding – also in later Daoist views – the newly buried person was thus still thought to be present. At this stage, with the two souls just starting to separate, the *qi* would still be active in the body and it might be possible that in this new state, removed from the sensory involvements and passions of the world, the person could still undertake the refinement of *qi* and transformation necessary to enhance life and attain a heavenly state. (2008, 35)

The written documents placed in the tomb with their son, were treasures then and now. There were texts on astronomy, politics, the Yi*jing* (Book of Changes), medicine, and exercise. Some texts were on bamboo, some on silk; all were carefully stacked in a lacquer case. For the time, it was a considerable compendium of important subjects for study and self-improvement. The tomb, interring the son and the self-improvement library, was closed. Some years later, the bodies of his father and mother were added and the tomb was permanently sealed in 168 BCE. It was not discovered until 1973.

When the collection of documents was found, there was quite a bit of excitement as they provided insight into a special period of cultural and scientific transition. Magical recipes, exorcisms, charms, and incantations are included in many of the medical texts. Donald Harper says,

> Significant spiritual and intellectual changes were clearly underway between the fourth and third centuries BCE. The changes produced a flowering of specialists in natural philosophy and occult knowledge in the third century BCE., as well as an explosion of *fang*-literature. I refer to the literature itself as '*fang literature*,' based on the significance of the concept of *fang* 方 (recipe) in defining natural philosophy and occult thought. (2009, 8)
>
> The Mawangdui medical texts belong to the third century BCE explosion. (2009, 39)

Some documents were well preserved and attention-getting, for example, a T-shaped silk painting on display in the Changsha Mawangdui Han Dynasty tombs exhibition. Other items were in poor condition, fragmented and enigmatic. One of these was a silk drawing (below), called the *Daoyintu* (Diagram of Guiding and Pulling). *Daoyin* is an ancient form of fitness and health activity. The Chinese word *tu* can be variously: map, chart, or diagram. We will use the term *Daoyintu* to refer to the painting on silk of the forty-four movements and *daoyin* as the generic word designating the energy and health cultivation practice.

Another trove of medical manuscripts, unearthed from a tomb at Jiangling, Zhangjianshan, included a text entitled *Yinshu* (The Pulling Book), which consisted of roughly 113 bamboo strips. Livia Kohn provides a detailed description of these exercises (2008, 41-61), while Vivienne Lo has published a full translation (2014). The *Yinshu* is considered "the earliest extant treatise on the Chinese tradition of *daoyin* (guiding and pulling), dating to the second century BCE" (Lo 2014, i). Text only, without pictures, it provides forty-one health exercises, but with scant relation to the *Daoyintu*. It is unfortunate that more instructions did not survive with the *Daoyintu* (see also App. 1).

The verbs "guiding" and "pulling" refer to guiding vital energy (*qi*) to desired locations and pulling out that which is painful, stale, toxic, or unwanted. (Harper 2009, 25). Part of the body of medical theory of the time was that spirits or demons caused illness. Theories of energy and blood flow were also becoming dominant at that time.

> By the third century BCE., ideas concerning the *mai* 脈 (vessels) filled with blood and *qi* 氣 (vapor) inside the body dominated physiological speculation; one definition of health was the maintenance of a constant supply of free-flowing blood and vapor in the vessels. (2009, 69)

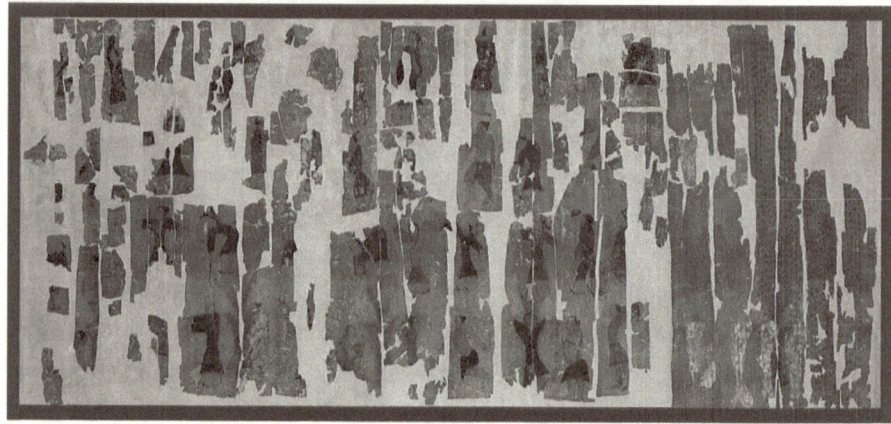

Fig 1. Original Mawangdui silk drawing.

As can be seen from the original silk drawing above, there was considerable damage. Thirteen of the figures and many of their names and functions were incomplete or missing. Over time, scholars and researchers pieced together information which was used to reconstruct images of the people practicing guiding and pulling or stretching. Figure 2 presents a reconstructed image of the original chart, that has appeared in many publications on this subject.

An Enigma at Mawangdui / 7

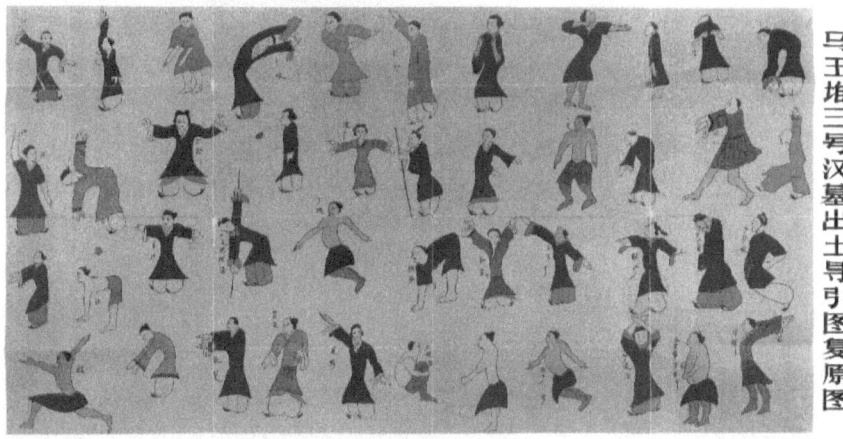

Fig. 2 Reconstructed image of the *Daoyintu*.

Although not included in the reconstruction, there are two sections of text to the right of the *daoyintu*.

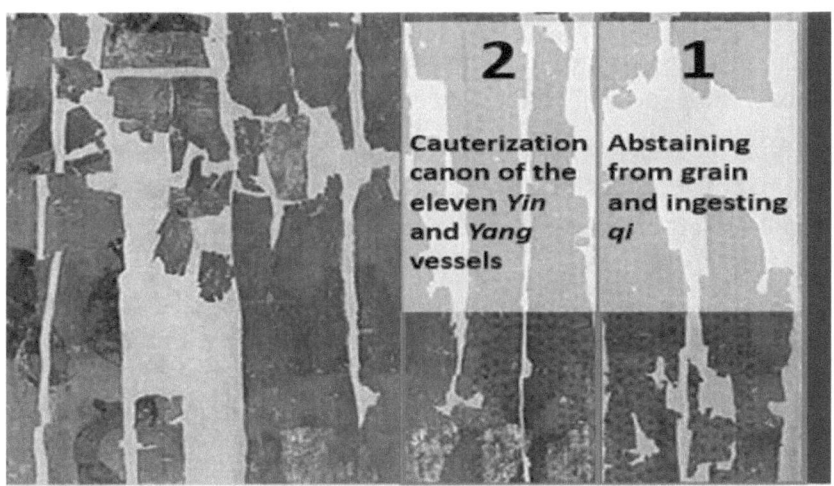

Fig. 3 Medical texts attached to the *Daoyintu*.

The text on the far right, referred to by Harper as MSII.A, is the *Quegu shiqi*, Eliminating Grain and Eating Vapor (or Abstaining from Grain and Ingesting Qi), that deals with breathing exercises. The text nearest to the images, referred to by Harper as MSI.B., is the *Yin yang shiyi mai jiujing yiben*, or Cauterization Canon of the Eleven Yin and Yang Vessels. (2009. 305-6). There could be connections between the two texts and the images, which doubtless warrant further research and discussion. Some aspects of breathing will be addressed in Chapter Three.

Analyzing the *Daoyintu*

The original *Daoyintu* silk drawing is incomplete, as are the instructions, and the figures are snapshots of movement, so the exact nature of the forty-four activities is open to interpretation. Since they were discovered in 1973, there have been a number of interpretive efforts to recreate the movements individually and as forms (combinations of movement). Some authors do not think the movements are in any discernable logical order. From inspection of the figures, and their surviving names, one can make the following observations:

Both men and women are doing the movements. They wear various types of clothing, possibly indicating that different classes of people did these movements.

Eight of the figures are bare chested. This could indicate the figures represent soldiers or laborers. Another interpretation is that figures shown without shirts indicate breathing patterns. That is, the creator of the chart used a protruding belly to indicate abdominal breathing and an indrawn belly to indicate reverse abdominal breathing.

At least four of the images indicate or imply making sounds. Others show tools or utensils. In two cases, poles are used. One object appears to be an apple. Several other objects have been variously interpreted as a bowl, disc, or bag.

Another key feature is that animal names are used at least nine times. The use of animals gives useful clues as to what kind of movement is likely intended, without accompanying instructions, although there is opportunity for interpretation. Vivienne Lo says,

> Consider, for example, the appeal to the imagination of animals in the context of *Daoyintu*, *Yinshu* and more generally throughout the culture of *daoyin*. Where a particular posture is given the name of an animal, there are immediate, commonly understood implications for the interpretation of that image with the body. But we cannot assume that we have grasped the full implications of the designation without questioning whether our understanding of a bear, monkey, crane or dragon is stunted by removal and distance. (Lo 2007, 84)

Animal movements indicate there was a shamanistic element to these healing activities and that a single movement or a number of movements could have been combined in a dance or *Daoyintu* form. As Catherine Despeux writes,

> In antiquity, *daoyin* movements evoked fluidity and were sometimes even used as dance. Judging by documents found at Mawangdui, Zhangjiashan [the *Yinshu*], and later, the practice of *daoyin* consisted mainly of isolated movements, but on occasion also formed a series of sequential movements constituting a real dance. One such series is described in the Zhangjiashan manuscript, *Yinshu*. However, dance in general was already present in the culture as a basic technique used by shamans, as described in the *Zhouli* (Rites of Zhou). (Despeux 2004, 61)

Daoyintu Images in Other Documents

There were most likely other copies of the *Daoyintu*, although none have been discovered. It is evident from a cursory review that *Daoyintu* images appeared in medical and exercise literature over the centuries. There are routines for specific ailments and general exercises in the *Yinshu* (Pulling Book), found in a manuscript dated to 186 BCE, two decades earlier than the *Daoyintu*.

In addition, the *Wuqinxi* (Five Animals' Frolics) of the physician Hua Tuo (2nd c. CE) could easily have drawn from the *Daoyintu* as four of the five animals (bear, tiger, monkey, and crane) appear in both. *Daoyintu*-like images appear in a Tang-dynasty book called *Qianjin yaofang* (Essential Prescriptions for Emergencies Worth a Thousand Pieces of Gold), in the *Baduan jin* (Eight Pieces of Brocade) as documented in the Southern Song dynasty, and in the so-called Forty-Nine Prescriptions of the Ming (see App. 1).

Over a third of the *Daoyintu* movements (i.e., #3, 4, 6, 9, 10, 15, 20, 21, 22, 25, 27, 28, 32, 39, 40, 42) appear also in other exercise routines, indicating that the chart has had a pervasive and lasting influence on Chinese health and energy practices over the centuries.

Naming Conventions

A number of the names and description of movements that did survive indicate that some were prescriptive for specific conditions, such as knee and ham (gluteus) pain. As stated above, many of the movements evoke the actions of animals and have names like "Bear Ramble" and "Crane Call." Where a name was decipherable from the manuscript, as interpreted by Donald Harper, it has been used with the associated figure. In some cases, the translations of Livia Kohn are used. Our teacher Hu Yang provided names for some of the other figures and we have used these. Where names were not given (or perhaps forgotten), the authors have provided ones they hope are descriptive and appropriate.

A Numbering System for the *Daoyintu* Movements

As the Chinese language is read in columns starting from right to left, one assumes the silk tapestry was meant to be read in the same way. Therefore, the figure in the top right corner of the silk tapestry is number 1. Having been taught the movements row by row starting at the top right-hand corner, we have therefore numbered the movements using the same convention. Thus, the figure just below #1 is #12 and the last figure in the lower left corner is #44. Both Donald Harper and Livia Kohn use this numbering convention, although Vivienne Lo uses a different convention.

After doing them for many years, our general feeling is that while some of these movements may seem quite simple and less refined than many modern energy exercises, they are very potent. When performed with a certain mind-set, one may have profound experiences. The animal movements are particularly powerful, as one emulates the animal, identifies with it, and forms a spiritual connection.

Chapter Two

Daoyintu Connections

This chapter is intended to provide some context for the *Daoyintu*, without going into a long discussion of Chinese history, Traditional Chinese Medicine, and Daoism, as there are many books on each subject.

The *Daoyintu* in History

According to Harper, the Mawangdui medical manuscripts represent a tradition of macrobiotic hygiene, that pre-dates the Yellow Emperor's classic, and may have been influenced by the *xian* (transcendent) cult of immortality. (2009, 7). Livia Kohn adds:

> All these texts are essentially part of the medical tradition. They were not in any major way related to Daoist philosophical speculation or the cult of immortality. (2008, 29)

Catherine Despeux states that *daoyin* practice has roots in shamanism:

> All in all, one can most clearly trace *daoyin* back to ancient techniques of ecstasy---to shamanism. The various traditions of daoyin all trace themselves back to rather well-known, albeit legendary, personages of old. There is the "Chinese Methuselah" Pengzu, there are the immortals Master Redpine and Wang Ziqiao, as well as the ancient master Ningfengzi. (1989, 237)

Daoyin is perhaps the earliest known Chinese term for energy cultivation. That energy is *qi*, which Harper translates as "vapor," and it is documented around the fourth century BCE (Harper 2014, 77). The term qigong, came into common usage much later and is now the term of art, but with many interpretations and connotations attached to it. We generally refrain from using the word qigong as we wish to focus on the older *daoyin* practices.

Readers may be quite familiar with the following subject matter, however, references are included, for those who wish to delve deeper.

Here are a few key events we believe are relevant. Any timeline of events in ancient Chinese history is problematic, as scholars can disagree considerably about dates. The following table provides an overview.

Table 1. The *Daoyintu* in History

Ca. 1000 BCE	*Yijing* (Book of Changes) (Huang 1998, xvi)
700-220 BCE	Classical period of Daoism (Wong 1997, 20)
551-479 BCE	Time of Confucius (Lynn 1999, 3)
500 BCE	Laozi's *Daodejing* (Cleary 1993, 2)
475-221 BCE	Breathing exercise inscribed on jade stone during Warring States period (Wu & Mao 1992, Illus. 1)
2nd c. BCE	*Huangdi neijing suwen* (The Yellow Emperor's Inner Classic, Simple Questions) (Veith 1949, 7-9)
186 BCE	*Yinshu* buried at Zhangjiashan
168 BCE	*Daoyintu* sealed in Mawangdui tomb (Harper 2009, 15)
25-220 CE	Physician Hua Tuo develops Five Animals' Frolics for longevity (14,) (Kohn 2008, 40)
400 CE or later	*Taiqing Daoyin yangsheng jing* (Great Clarity Scripture of Healing Exercises and Nourishing Life, in Daoist Canon) (Despeux 1989, 230)
1368-1644	Term qigong first mentioned in a written document (Ming Dynasty). (Cohen 1997, 13)

Sui dynasty 581-618	*Yangsheng fang daoyin fa* (The *Yangsheng* Recipes: The *Daoyin* Methods) in *Zhubing yuanhou lun* (Treatise on the Origins and Symptoms of Medical Disorders) (Yang 2018, 22)
1947	Medical qigong for health introduced by Liu Guizhen (Johnson 2005, 13)
1973	*Daoyintu* discovered with other manuscripts and materials in the Mawangdui tomb (Harper 2009, 25)

Traditional Chinese Medicine

Chinese physicians treat the human body as an integral system of interrelated networks with different physiological functions. The system uses energy pathways to link the organs and other human systems into a unified whole.

> In Chinese medicine, health is the ability of an organism to respond appropriately to a wide variety of challenges in a way that insures maintaining equilibrium and integrity. Disease represents a failure to adapt to challenge, a disruption of the overall equilibrium, a rent in the fabric of the organism. (Beinfeld and Korngold 1991, 36)

The subject is complex, so we will touch on a few selected aspects.

Yin and yang are "convenient symbols to represent two opposing yet complimentary aspects in medicine and all other fields" (Kit 2002, 33). A deficiency, or an excess of either one can cause disease. Essentially, good health is maintaining yin and yang in harmony.

Next, the five phases (*wuxing*) are wood, fire, earth, metal, and water. They represent processes that interact continuously. Over time, they became associated with organs, emotions and a host of other things that are too complex to discuss in detail here. Basically, the five phases need to be kept in balance for optimal health (Maciocia 1989, 21-22; see also App. 2).

The triple heater, also known as triple warmer or burner (*sanjiao*), marks three distinct energy processing centers in the torso: an upper in the lung area, a middle one in the upper abdomen, and one in its lower section. Functionally, these areas contain the organs of breathing, activities of food processing, and two of the three energy centers that are known as cinnabar or elixir fields, *dantian* in Chinese. Air and food are converted to qi in these areas, which is further stored in them.

The lower of the three is located three finger-widths below the navel; the middle field is found in the area of the sternum, roughly at the nipple line; and the upper one resides in the center of the head, accessible by mentally moving inward from between the eyebrows.

> Since people may get the warm sensation in different parts of the body there are diverse opinions about the location of Dan Tien. However, it is accepted that there are three *dantian* regions: upper, middle, and lower *dan-tian*. According to traditional Chinese medicine, the "three treasures" in the body—*jing*, *qi*, and *shen*—are stored in the lower, middle, and upper elixir field respectively. (Cen 1996. 30)

Within this geography, the body also contains Three Treasures (*sanbao*). Giovanni Maciocia, writes, "One of the most important characteristics of Chinese medicine is the close integration of body and mind, which is highlighted by the close integration of essence, *qi*, and spirit (mind), called the Three Treasures" (1989, 69). There are various interpretations of the three. Essence (*jing*) is commonly interpreted as the vital power of life or sexual energy. It is located in the lower elixir field. "This pre-heaven essence is what determines each person's basic constitutional make-up, strength and vitality. It is what makes the individual unique" (Maciocia 1989, 44).

Qi, sometimes also called post-heaven essence, is vital energy from many sources, including breathing, eating, drinking, and gathering. This *qi* is located in the middle elixir field, and it affects interactions between the five phases, organs, and emotions.

Shen is defined as spirit or mind. It is associated with the heart-mind and located in the upper elixir field. "Of all the organs, the Mind is most closely related to the Heart, which is said to be the Mind's residence." He goes on to say, "if the Mind is disturbed by emotional stress, becoming unhappy, depressed, anxious or unstable it will definitely affect *qi* or essence, or both" (Maciocia 1989, 69).

Another description of *shen*, which is particularly appealing to us, is that of Daoist master Zhao Bichen: "*Shen* is spiritual and psychic energy, the divine part of the being, whose nature is essentially luminous." (Despeux 1979, 55).

Daoism and Primordial Emptiness

Although *daoyin* was not originally a Daoist practice, the authors have found a Daoist perspective was especially helpful to awaken our creativity and enhance our ability to bring the *Daoyintu* images to life.

The word "Dao" literally means "way" or "road."

> The original Dao is conceived of supreme emptiness, from which the One, which is none other than primordial breath, emanates. This gives birth to the two, embodied by the two vital breaths of yin and yang. By their interaction, yang as the active force, and yin, as receptive softness, govern the multiple vital breaths that animate the ten thousand existents of the created world. (Cheng 1994, 50)

There are key Daoist concepts that influence our practice: nonaction, the uncarved block, and virtue. To begin, nonaction (*wuwei*) has been variously defined as inaction, being passive, and letting go. Alan Watts interprets it as not forcing things (1975, 76). We like this definition. We also like the idea of letting go.

The uncarved block (*pu*) encourages people to look deeply and find what is hidden within. One may reminisce on the often-told story of the artist who found a precious stone and sculpted his most esthetic creation. When asked how he created such a beautiful piece, the sculptor replied, "The statue was always there. It was only waiting for someone to bring it to life." Holmes Welch notes that the *Daodejing* in places also uses the word "simplicity" (*su*) to express the same idea. *Su* literally means raw silk, i.e., that which has not been dyed nor painted (Welch 1966, 35).

Virtue *(de)* is not a simple concept. Alan Watts defines it as a concept that is broader than moral virtue. "It is rather as when we speak of the healing virtues of a plant, having the connotation of power or even magic, when magic refers to wonderful and felicitous events which come about spontaneously" (Watts 1975, 107). It manifests best after quieting the mind and excluding the outside world: "Your own *de* is infinite and, when you return to awareness of the physical world, this infinite *de*, which is more than the effectiveness of outward inaction and more than the power of intuitive understanding, will protect you from all harm to the end of your days" (Welch 1966, 84).

We think that the best definition of virtue in the context of this book is that of an intuitive understanding that manifests positive intentions, that is, a kind of enlightened power.

The Enigma of the *Daoyintu*

The *Daoyintu* images are like shadows on a wall. Those that are complete provide some information about how to perform particular movements, but with limited instructions. They are enigmatic. A number of images, moreover, are so incomplete that they are less than shadows; they can be considered *su*, very open to creative interpretation.

> And art is always symbolic: it always expresses more than its explicit content. Since both the cultural experiences and symbolic systems vary from one people to another, artistic expression varies widely. With art, as in life, the basic natural man is submerged in the cultural circumstance in which it appears. (Goldschmidt 1960, 581)

Every society, every person, has the urge to create something. The *Daoyintu* movements were created by a physician/shaman for the purpose of health. The images that portray these health concepts are art in themselves and therefore subject to interpretation and free expression.

Chapter Three

Practice Guidelines

As you start to practice these movements there are a number of things to keep in mind. First, the various exercises are complementary health practices that serve to augment treatment you may already be receiving from a physician.

Second, always seek medical advice from your doctor before starting any kind of new physical activity. Use common sense. If a movement or activity causes any pain, stop doing it. It is advisable to wait at least an hour (preferably two) after eating before practicing *Daoyintu*.

Third, when you are finished doing a set of movements, make a point of meditating in a seated or lying position afterwards for ten to fifteen minutes or more. Wait at least an hour after your practice before eating, but drinking water or tea is fine.

Here are more specific guidelines, arranged under distinct headings.

Physical/Mechanical

We suggest that you initially consider these *Daoyintu* activities as simple stretches; starting slowly and using common sense, to get comfortable with the movements and breathing patterns. While it is natural to feel your muscles, ligaments, and tendons while stretching, it is also important to focus on your joints, even to the point of meditating or moving *qi* to them.

No one will do the movements in exactly the same way. Anyone who teaches taiji quan or qigong knows that each person's mind and body reproduce a posture or set of movements in ways that are uniquely theirs, no matter how many times you repeat or "correct" them. If we are honest with ourselves, we all do personal approximations of what we are taught. The movements should be as structurally correct as you can make them; they should never hurt; and after a time, they should feel "right" to you.

Note which of the *Daoyintu* movements you really like and which ones, if any, don't appeal to you. One of the authors had a Marine Corps student who remarked that you should do more of the exercises that you don't like. Take that approach if it works for you. We have found, over time, that some movements fall out of favor and others take their place.

How fast and forcefully should you perform these *Daoyintu* movements? Do each of them slowly to begin with. Some of the images communicate that a movement could be forceful, to assist in pulling a disease. We have given some advice with certain images, but you can perform each movement as slowly, or fast, as you wish according to your personal rhythm. How many times should you perform these movements? As a general rule, repeat three to nine times, although you should not be limited by this guideline if you feel like doing more repetitions of a given movement, then do so.

Breathing

Breathing is one of the simplest things we do, usually without thinking much about it. Many books have been written about breathing techniques, the main ones being: normal breathing, abdominal breathing, reverse abdominal breathing, and fetal breathing. Use of these techniques is a matter of practitioner's choice.

First is the so-called normal, unconscious breathing, which has been described as "somewhat superficial" by Hu Bin (1982). It uses mainly the chest muscles and throat. For many people who breathe in this manner, the inhalations and exhalations are shallow and relatively quick. An exercise we use in beginning meditation classes is to count the number of times you do a complete inhale and exhale in 60 seconds. Quite a few people take ten or more breaths per minute in their normal breathing. It is very possible to reduce the number of breaths per minute with practice.

Second is abdominal breathing. This involves relaxing the abdominal muscles as you inhale (thus causing the abdomen to protrude) and pushing in with your abdominal muscles as you exhale. In this fuller breathing process, muscles in both the chest and abdomen are employed. More oxygen is brought into the body and there is a greater exhalation of stale air from the lungs. Abdominal breathing is one technique used during energy practice such as *daoyin*, qigong, or yoga; it is a gentler, more relaxing means of acquiring *qi*, and is viewed by some as being less efficient than reverse abdominal breathing for that purpose.

Third is reverse abdominal breathing, which as the name indicates, involves pulling your abdominal muscles in on inhalation and relaxing the abdominal muscles on exhalation. This takes some practice and effort to do. Especially in the beginning one can employ too much muscular effort; therefore, one needs to condition the "breathing muscles" and be cautious about overly exerting oneself. Reverse abdominal breathing is another technique used during energy practice and it has the added feature of forcing *qi* into the upper body cavity. In general, reverse abdominal breathing is used for *qi* application in martial arts and acquiring large amounts of *qi* for healing.

Fourth is fetal breathing, pre-natal breathing or embryo respiration. This last is the Daoist term for "breathing like a child in the womb" (Welch 1957, 108). This implies naturalness in breathing, that is, thought and intention free. You can think of it as a kind of innocence of breathing. It is based on ancient observations, confirmed by modern medical science, that a fetus in the womb does not breathe itself, but receives nurture and oxygen through the umbilicus. Fetal breathing is seen as breathing without any effort, or sound. It is said the ultimate goal of Daoist breathing practice is to breathe without breath. This is an advanced technique, and while the goal of breathing naturally and without thought can be achieved to one degree or another, the most advanced forms may be beyond some of us.

One of the authors uses abdominal breathing and the other uses reverse abdominal breathing. We recommend that you use abdominal breathing to start.

We should all strive to breathe better; more deeply on inhalation and exhalation, while using our abdominal muscles in a relaxed way. This is true whether you are breathing "normally," abdominally, or using the reverse abdominal method. If you are new to breathing methods, you should practice a method of breathing without any distractions or movements. In other words, first develop your breathing techniques in stillness or meditation and then apply them to *Dao* yin and other energy-cultivating movements. The *Daoyintu* figure #19 depicts a straightforward breathing exercise that would be a good place to start breathing practice.

Sounds

You will naturally make sounds while performing many of these movements. The more emphatic movements will likely generate forceful sounds. Where appropriate, we have suggested specific sounds to accompany them. The *Quegu shiqi* text, mentioned in Chapter two, refers to certain healing sounds made during exhalation, those sounds being *xu*, *chui,* and *hu*. Although instructions are not available in the text, Harper states that another medical document, the *Yinshu*, describes using a *xu* exhalation for heat, *chui* exhalation for dampness, and *hu* exhalation for dryness (2009, 305-06).

Approximately, the sound *xu* is "shoe," *chui* is "shway" and *hu* is "hoo." These sounds, as well as other sounds used in energy healing regimes, or your own natural sounds, could certainly be voiced in your *Daoyintu* practice.

Qi

When you are comfortable and relaxed with the movements and your breathing, start to focus on the flow of your *qi*, the underground river that runs through us all. Rather than attempting to direct it, try to feel where each of these special movements causes your *qi* to go and notice any sensations. We have provided a generalized description of how we feel energy during the movements.

In chapter 2, we described that the Three Treasures are pre-heaven essence (*jing*), post-heaven energy (*qi*), and the heart-mind (*shen*). Their complex interplay makes us who we are: genetically, physically, energetically, and emotionally. When we practice the exercises outlined in the *Daoyintu*, we naturally pay close attention to the flow of *qi*, but we should not neglect these other aspects. We use the term, "stale essence," referring to used breath, turbid *qi*, disease, and negative emotions. "Fresh essence" signals new breath, external *qi*, and positive emotions in healthy balance.

Guiding and Pulling

The authors find it helpful to think of the *Daoyintu* energetic process in terms of "guiding and pulling out, then pulling and guiding in." The "guiding and pulling out" concerns more than just your *qi*. It is the process of accumulating stale essence, internally guiding and pulling it to points where it can exit your body, then releasing it through actions such as exhalation, extending limbs, shaking, and flicking. *Daoyintu* #8 and 9 are examples of movements that expel stale essence through your extended limbs, including fingers and toes. As your extended limbs return to neutral position, you are pulling in fresh essence.

There is a point where you can feel an external pulling of unwanted essence from your extremities. This leaves a space, or vacuum, that needs to be refilled and brought back into balance. As part of the rebalancing process, the pulling out reverses direction and becomes a pulling in. The second pulling and guiding in fills you up with fresh essence and moves it to where you want it, for example, an elixir field, organ, or other location that is meaningful to you. Although this step-by-step description may seem cumbersome, with practice, the actual process becomes easy and natural. Of course, it is your option to add guiding and pulling to your energy practice.

Spiritual/Emotional

"It is when emotions are prolonged, intense, repressed or not acknowledged that they become a cause of an imbalance of a person's *qi*" (Hicks and Mole 2007, 27).

Traditionally, negative emotions are used in diagnosis and treatment by trained practitioners. This is an approach which is due, in part, to the ethically oriented Confucian influences upon Chinese medicine. (Maciocia 2009, 314-40). We note this emphasis on negative emotions, but suggest to overly focus on them may be counter-productive to self-improvement. Instead, we suggest the approach of expelling negative emotions, and replacing them with positive emotions as preparation for personal reflection on self-care.

Having love in one's life is a source of positive emotions, and this concept was written about more than 1500 years ago.

> One of the most interesting discussions, both theoretically and therapeutically, can be found in the writings of the greatest physician of the Tang Dynasty, Sun Simiao (590-682 CE). Some of his notions have an astonishingly modern ring, and it is worth transmitting his insight: people suffer illness because they do not have love in their life and are not cherished. (Kaptchuk 2000, 159)

Smiling into one's self, the elixir fields, and the organs is a powerful practice and an effective step toward self-love.

You should be aware of your negative emotions, but do not dwell on them as you guide and pull them out. Embrace positive emotions and pull and guide them in. Unburdening yourself and filling up with positive emotions are practices that form a key part of doing *Daoyintu* exercises. Movement #5 is an example of this process that involves replacing grief with joy.

Some movements are especially suited for meditation and spiritual experiences that bring you in tune with nature or even the cosmos. Individual experiences may vary greatly. It is possible you may have a connection with the spirit of one or more animals while doing certain *Daoyintu* movements. In ancient Chinese culture, shamans had a spiritual relationship with certain animals.

> But we must not forget that the relations between the shaman (and, indeed, "primitive man" in general) and animals are spiritual in nature and of a mystical intensity that a modern, desacralized mentality finds it difficult to imagine. (Eliade 2004, 459)

One does not need to be a shaman to imitate one of the *Daoyintu* animal movements and feel a connection that is both interesting and enjoyable. You can try #20 and 25 to experience such a connection.

Opening the Practice

We suggest that you begin each movement from the *Wuji* stance. The term *wuji* has been translated in many ways, but we prefer to follow the definition by Tsung-Hwa Jou: "Ancient Chinese philosophers called the void and boundless state that prevailed before the world was created and from which the universe was formed Wu-Chi [Wuji] or the ultimate nothingness" (2001, 87).

The initial stance, then, should be as balanced and neutral as possible before you enter the dynamic state of creation. The instructions are as follows:

---

1. Start with your feet shoulder distance apart, with feet flat on the ground.
2. Bend your knees slightly.
3. Allow your center of gravity to sink (imagine you are starting to sit down on a tall stool).
4. Your arms should hang slightly away from your torso.
5. Relax your shoulders.
6. Tuck your chin in slightly.
7. Place your tongue on the roof of your mouth.
8. Feel your spine elongate as your head is lifted as though pulled by a string.

These standing posture guidelines can easily be adapted for a person who is seated. In either case, your body should feel relaxed; also, having a slight smile on your face wouldn't hurt.

Chapter Four

Movements 1 through 11

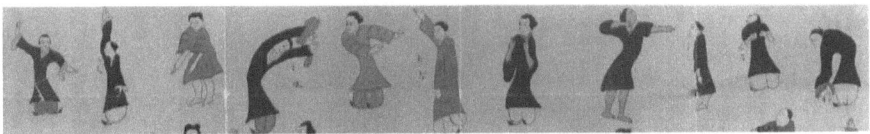

Fig. 4: The top row of *Daoyintu*.

The first row presents eleven movements, showing seven figures in legible condition, so that one can determine the positions of arms and legs. #2, 6, 7, and 9 are artist's extrapolations from the damaged original.

In general, the underlying focus of these first movements is on preparatory stretches and loosening activities (#1, 4, 6, 7, 11). There are also self-massages (#2 and 5) and some examples of pulling stale essence (#1, 2, 5, 6, 7, 8, 9, and 10). Sounds are implied in #2. After a slow warmup, #7, 8, 9, and 10 can be done forcefully to expel stale essence.

The authors have used three sources for the translation of the names of *Daoyintu* movements. (H) = Harper 2009; (K) = Kohn 2008; (Y) = Madam Hu Yang. Where no name was indicated, we have provided one, marked (A) = authors.

26 / Chapter Four

1. Opening to Heaven and Earth (A)

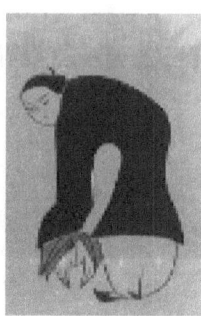

Action: Opens the body to prepare for muscular and energetic activity.
Muscles: Diaphragm, back, gluteus, hamstrings, calves.
Joints: Shoulders, hips, and spine.
Qi Flow: Rising from the feet to the fingertips, then down into the earth. As the spine opens up, one may feel energy strongly in the back.
Spiritual-Emotional: Opening to self, lightness, and release.
Instructions: 1. Stand relaxed with feet comfortably apart.   2. Inhale as you raise both arms to the sides and over your head. Feel your spine elongate.   3. Bring your arms down slowly and bend your neck forward, feeling your cervical vertebrae opening.   4. Exhale and slowly bend forward at the waist to feel your thoracic vertebrae opening. Repeat Steps 2 through 4 several times until you feel quite stretched and open.   5. This time, as you raise your arms over your head, guide and pull stale essence to your fingertips and release it above you. Pull and guide fresh essence into yourself.   6. As your fingertips near the earth, allow stale essence to be pulled from your body into the earth. (You may bend your knees as much as you wish).

7. Inhale as you slowly straighten, pulling fresh essence into your body, while bringing your crossed wrists up to the lower elixir field (scooping up). Optionally, do not cross your wrists.
8. As you raise both arms again, guide and pull stale essence to your fingertips and release into the sky.
9. Pull in fresh essence from above and below as you continue opening to heaven and earth.

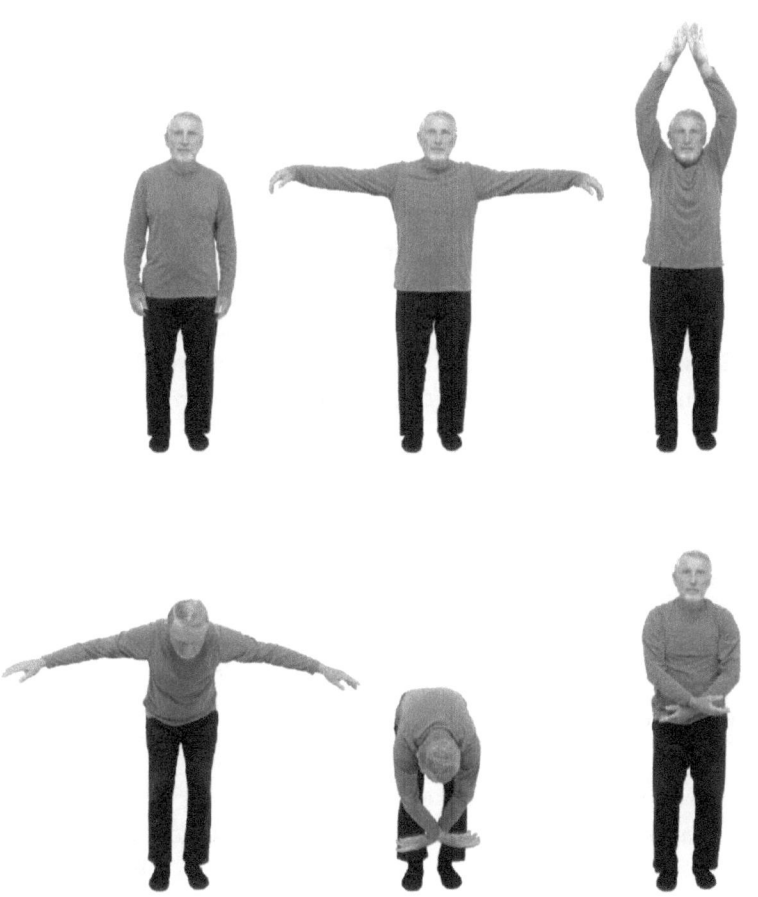

2. Pulling Stale Essence (A)

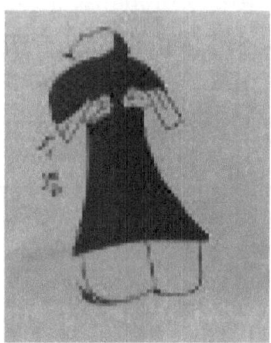

Actions: Opens the lungs, clears out stale essence, massages kidneys, and muscles of the back.
Muscles: Shoulders, back and pectorals.
Joints: neck, arms, shoulders, spine and hips.
Qi Flow: Stale essence is gathered from the body, then expelled with the breath. Kidneys are activated to bring fresh *qi* to the lungs.
Spiritual-Emotional: Feeling of release, clearing, and renewal.
Instructions: 1. Your feet are comfortably apart. Carefully tilt your head back.   2. Rub your kidneys to activate them and moisten your lungs.   3. Lightly strike your back muscles with your fists, avoiding your kidneys and spine. Find your comfortable pressure.   4. Move your hands up and down your back as far as you can reach.   5. Expel air and guide stale essence through your mouth with a sensation of the "HAAAH" sound being pulled out of you. You may optionally use healing sounds: "shoe," "shway," and "hoo."   6. When you feel you have sufficiently expelled stale essence, take more breaths with the purpose of pulling in fresh essence and guide it where you want it to go.

Movements 1 through 11 / 29

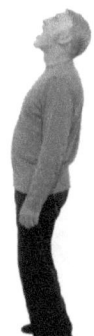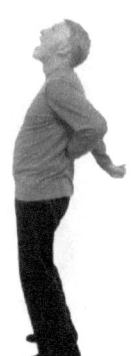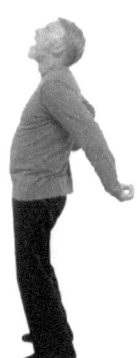

3. Twisting the Torso (Y)

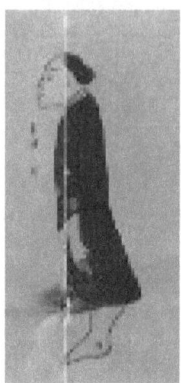

Actions: Loosens the torso; moves and massages the organs.
Muscles: Waist, hips, abdominals.
Joints: Hips, knees, spine.
Qi Flow: Expanding from the organs and torso to the upper and lower extremities. You may also feel energy flow back and forth along your hips.
Spiritual-Emotional: Comforting, relaxing.
Instructions: 　1.　Feet shoulder-width apart or closer. 　2.　Align your perineum, your spine, and the top of your head on one vertical axis. 　3.　Slowly turn your torso and head from left to right with arms by your sides. 　4.　Turn your torso a bit faster and let both arms swing loosely. 　5.　Movement comes from the waist as arms impact the front and back of your torso and massage internal organs: kidneys, liver, and spleen. 　6.　Be still. Guide and pull stale essence from your organs. 　7.　Pull and guide fresh essence into your body from head to toes.

Movements 1 through 11 / 31

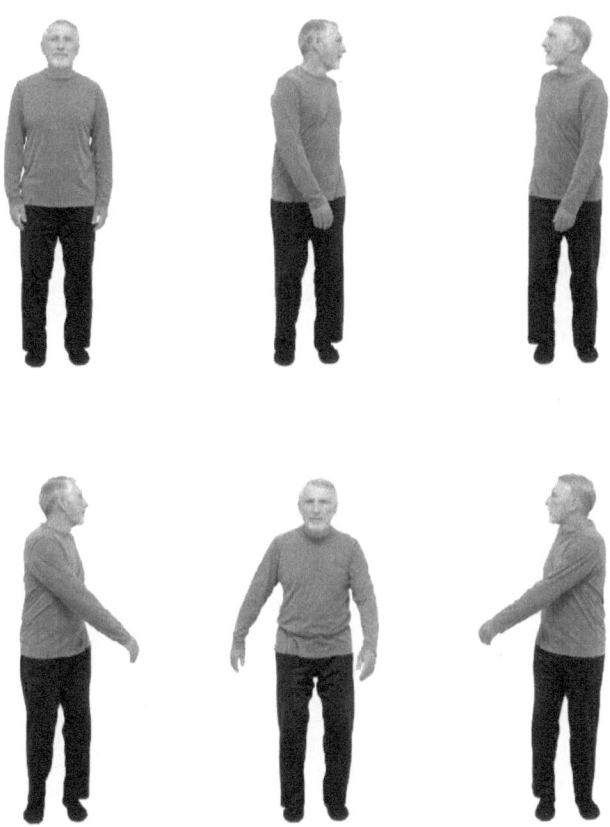

4. Shooting Arrow (Y)

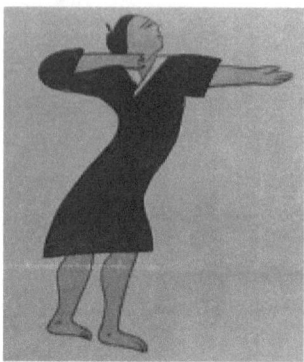

Actions: Stretching, focusing attention, activates the Liver, inducing brightness in the eyes.
Muscles: Shoulders, arms, upper back, chest, legs.
Joints: Shoulders, elbows, wrists, knees.
Qi Flow: Rising to shoulders, arms, and fingertips, then sinking to lower elixir field.
Spiritual-Emotional: Mental focus, imagination, a feeling of joy at "arrow" release, eyes focus your spirit.
Instructions: 1. Horse Stance with feet wide, or feet shoulder-width apart. 2. Cross wrists in front of chest. If desired, step left. 3. Turn waist to the left. Inhale, as you draw back an imaginary bowstring with your right hand while extending your left hand with index finger straight and thumb pointing to the right. Guide stale essence into the imaginary arrow. 4. Focus on a real or imagined target. Exhale, and allow the fingers of the right hand to relax, releasing the bowstring. Breathe in fresh essence. 5. Turn waist to the right and draw back the bowstring with your left hand, shooting to your right. You can repeat multiple shots in each direction.

Movements 1 through 11 / 33

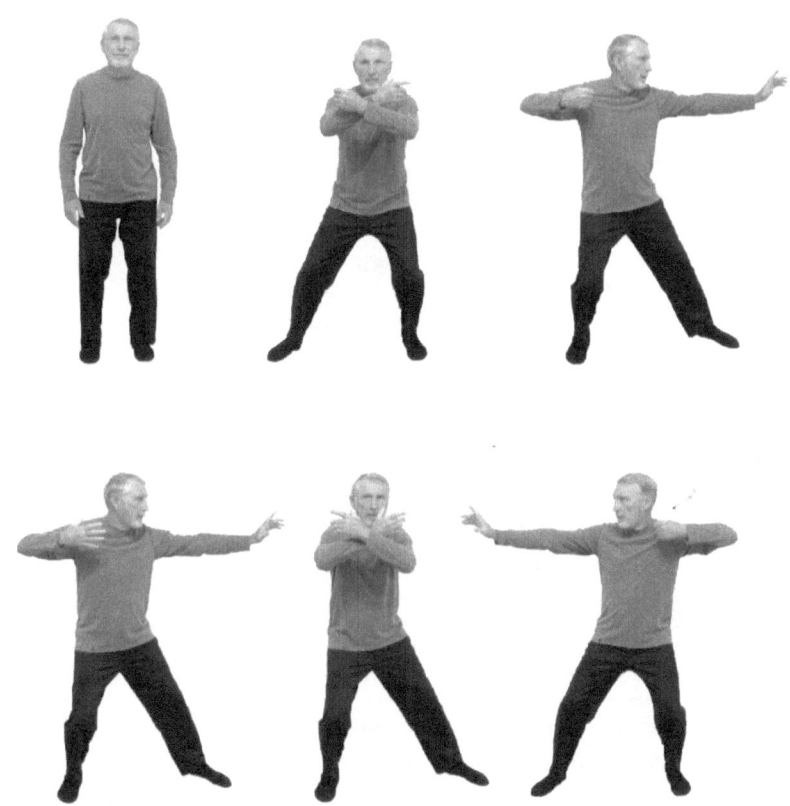

5. Gently Tapping Middle Palace and Cloud Gate (A)

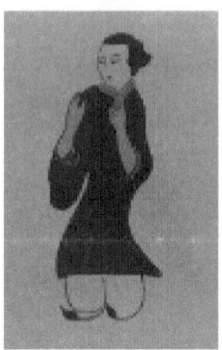

Actions: Loosening and self-massage of Lung 1 and 2: Zhongfu, the Middle Mansion, aka Central Treasury, below the clavicle; and Yunmen, Cloud Gate, above Zhongfu.
Muscles: Chest, shoulders, biceps, triceps.
Joints: Shoulders, elbows.
Qi Flow: Rising to chest and back, sinking back to the lower elixir field. Stale essence is guided to chest and pulled from the points Lung 1 and 2.
Spiritual-Emotional: Clearing anxiety or grief, release.
Instructions: 1. Feet shoulder-width apart, form "beaks" by placing fingers together with thumb. 2. Elbows down in front of chest. 3. Using short strokes, tap area where your shoulder meets your chest (Lung 1 and 2). Use your beaks to activate those points. 4. Left hand to left chest and right to right, or you can cross over with left hand to right shoulder, and right hand to left shoulder. 5. Now, be still. Use your beaks, as you exhale, to pull out the stale essence (especially the emotion of grief). 6. Inhale to pull fresh essence, including joy, into Lung 1 and 2 with your breath.

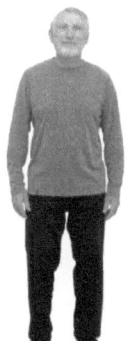 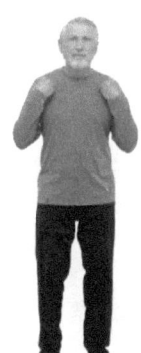 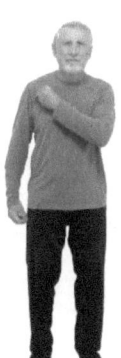 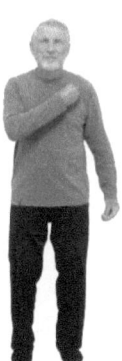

6. Snapping Yin (H)

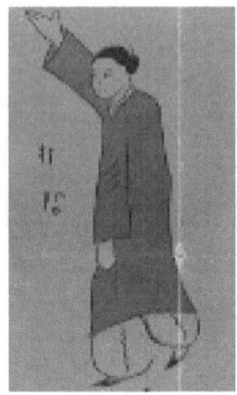

Actions: Stretch, balance, and exchange energy.
Muscles: Thighs, hamstrings, shoulders, back.
Joints: Hips, knees, ankles, shoulders, wrists.
Qi Flow: Rising up the back to shoulders, arms, and fingertips, where stale essence is pulled from the hands. Next, fresh essence is pulled in and guided back to the lower elixir field and down the legs to the toes.
Spiritual-Emotional: Centering, balancing, focusing attention within.
Instructions: 1. Feet shoulder-width apart, let your *Mingmen* (Gate of Life) sink down. This point is GV-4, in the lower back near kidneys). 2. Raise your right palm as you also lift your left leg to a comfortable level. Hold the position, if possible. 3. Feel stale essence move and be pulled out through hands and feet. 4. Fresh essence is pulled and guided to the lower elixir field as you drop your right hand and left leg. 5. Repeat on other side with left palm and right leg. Hold. 6. You may also feel stale essence be pulled out of your *Mingmen* and fresh essence be pulled in.

Movements 1 through 11

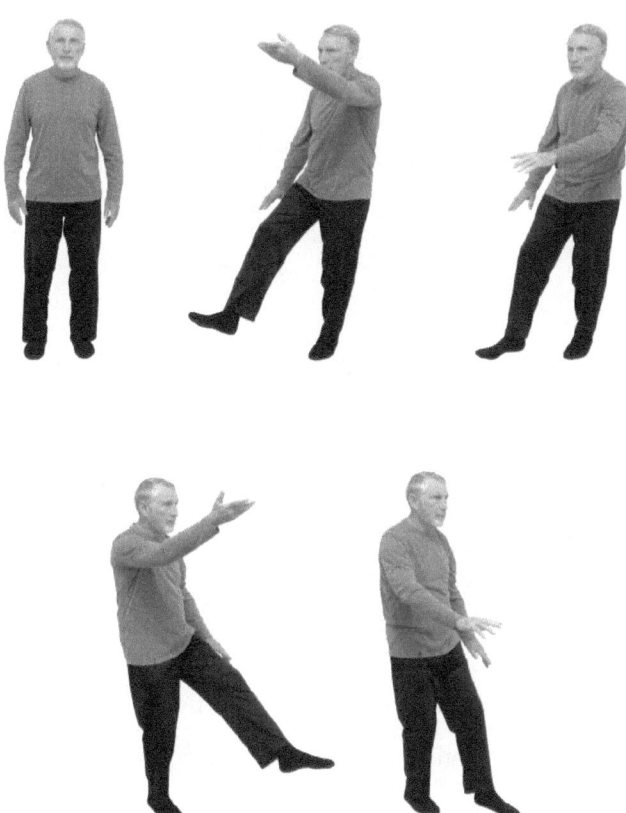

7. Swirling *Qi* from Earth to Sky (A)

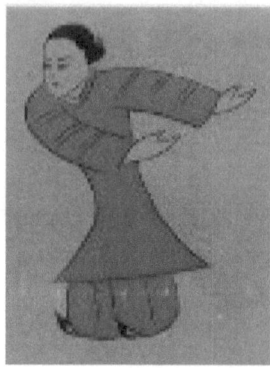

Actions: Stretching, twisting, releasing.
Muscles: Back, shoulders, torso, hamstrings.
Joints: Neck, hips, shoulders.
Qi Flow: Stale essence is guided from the lower elixir field to the shoulders, arms, and hands, where it is pulled out and exchanged for fresh essence, then guided back to the lower elixir field.
Spiritual-Emotional: Comforting, connecting with earth, uplifting, release.
Instructions: 1. Feet shoulder-width apart and raise both arms to your left. 2. Your eyes follow your hands throughout the movement. 3. Bend forward, as though to brush your toes with your fingertips. You may bend less deeply, if desired. 4. Let both arms swing through from left to right, like a pendulum. 5. Turn your head to watch your hands as they rise to the right. Pause. Feel stale essence being pulled out and replaced. 6. Bend forward again letting arms swing down to knee level and up to the left. Pause. Feel stale essence pulled out and replaced.

Movements 1 through 11 / 39

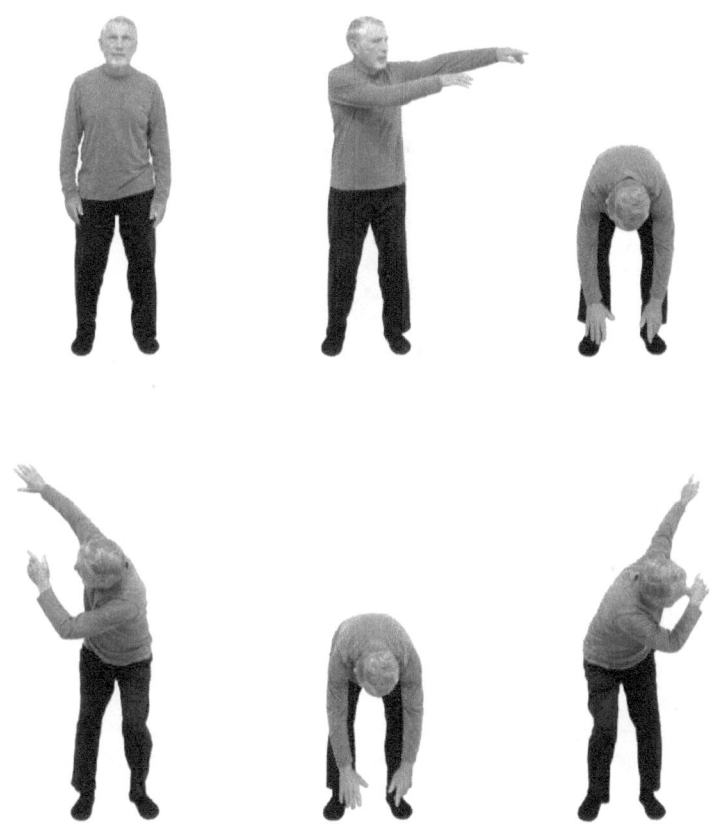

8. Praying Mantis (H)

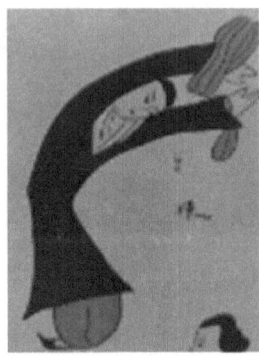

Actions: Stretching, twisting, organ massage.
Muscles: Back, intercostals, core, shoulders, arms, legs.
Joints: Hips, shoulders, elbows, knees.
Qi Flow: Guided up back from the lower elixir field to arms and hands, where it is pulled out, replaced by pulling in fresh essence that is guided back to the elixir field.
Spiritual-Emotional: Imagination, visualizing a mantis striking, and letting go.
Instructions: 1. Feet shoulder-width apart, fingers touching thumbs, wrists relaxed in front of chest with elbows down. 2. Thrust arms and hands up and out to the left upper left side (10 o'clock) while you simultaneously move your left foot about 45 degrees to the left and point your left toes to touch the ground. 3. Curl your back as you lift your rib cage. 4. You may extend your fingers to feel stale essence being pulled out. 5. As you bring your wrists back in front of your chest, feel fresh essence being pulled in.

6. Repeat the movement to the right.

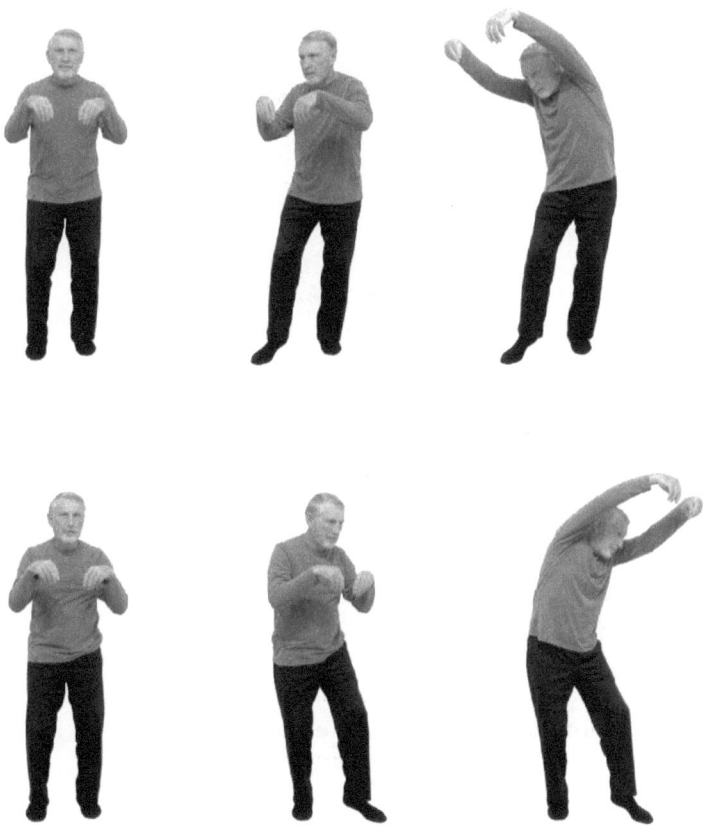

42 / Chapter Four

9. Thrusting Palms (Y)

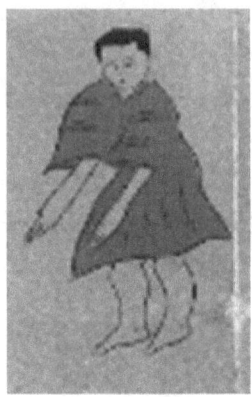

Actions: Stretching, vibrating.
Muscles: Waist, back, chest, shoulders, limbs.
Joints: Hips, spine, shoulders.
Qi Flow: Stale essence is guided from the body to the shoulders and pulled from the fingertips. Fresh essence is pulled in and guided back to the lower elixir field.
Spiritual-Emotional: deliberate, or emphatic release.
Instructions: 1. Feet shoulder-width apart, elbows hanging comfortably by your sides, with palms facing up. Guide stale essence to your shoulders. 2. Bend forward at the waist and thrust your arms forward, with palms still up, allowing stale essence to be pulled from your fingertips. Make a healing sound as you exhale. 3. Straighten up, as you pull in fresh essence, guide it to the lower elixir field and repeat. 4. Start very slowly; you may increase speed of thrusts if you wish but don't lose the feeling of the guiding and pulling process.

Movements 1 through 11 / 43

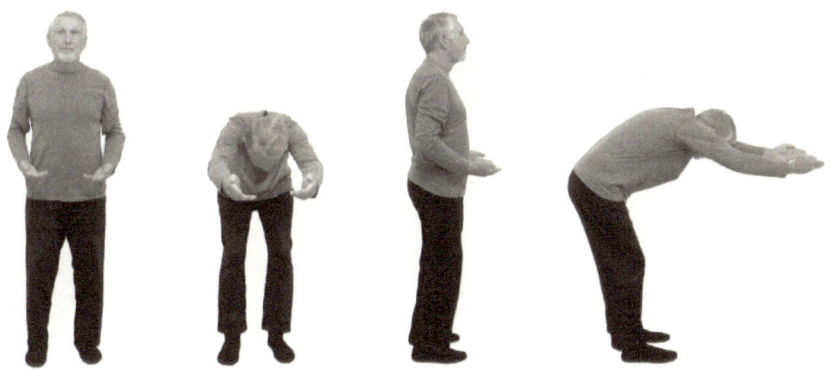

10. Limbs Dropping (H)

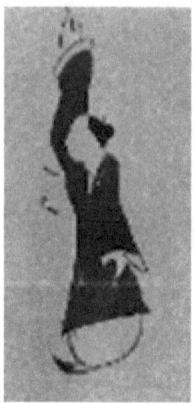

Actions: Stretching, releasing muscles and expelling stale essence through the action of your dropping arm.
Muscles: Back, shoulders, arms, upper back, chest.
Joints: Shoulders and knees
Qi Flow: Guided to chest, shoulders, arms, and fingertips, as one raises the limb. As the limb drops, stale essence is pulled out. Fresh essence is pulled in and guided to the lower elixir field through the lowered limb.
Spiritual-Emotional: Connecting heaven and earth, you are yin and yang in resonance.
Instructions: 1. Lift right arm straight up over your shoulder, left arm is pulled back slightly (you should feel comfortable tension in your pectoral muscles). Guide stale essence to your right arm and hand. Hold the position momentarily to feel it gathering. 2. Allow your right arm to drop naturally forward and down as you exhale. Your knees bend and your left arm hangs naturally down. Pause, to feel stale essence release into the earth, then pull in fresh essence.

3. Straighten your legs as you lift your left arm straight up and your right arm is pulled back slightly. Guide stale essence to your left arm and hand. Hold the position momentarily to feel it gathering.

4. Allow your left arm to drop naturally forward and down as you exhale. Your knees bend and your right arm hangs naturally down. Pause, to release stale essence into the earth, then pull in fresh essence.

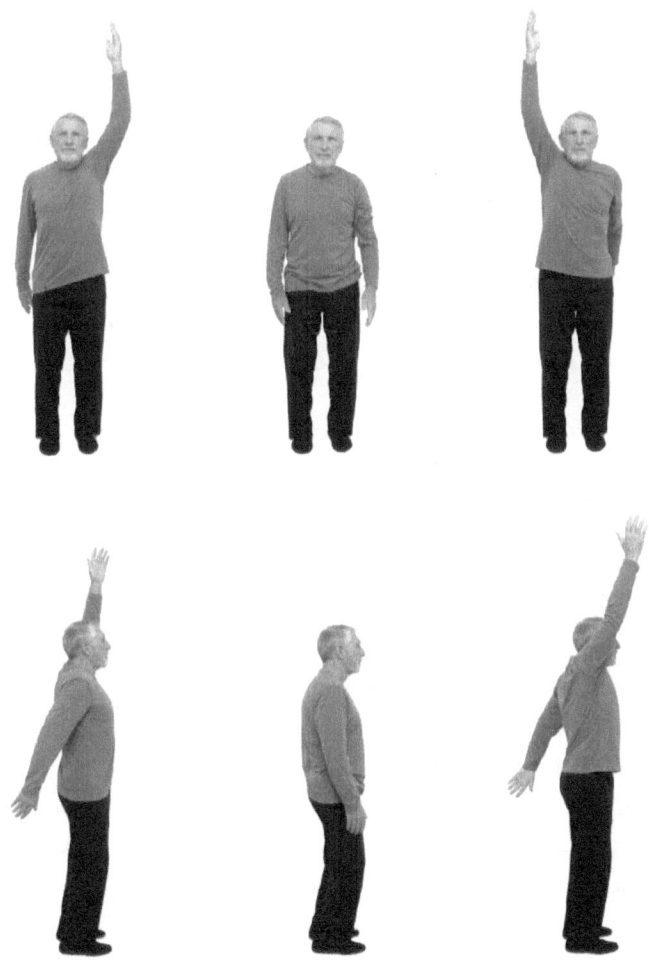

46 / Chapter Four

11. Expanding into the Cosmos (A)

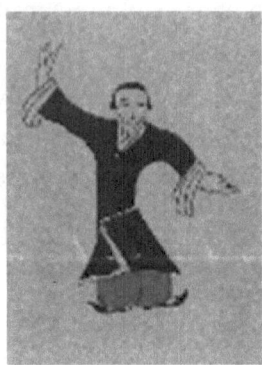

Actions: Stretching, twisting, full body integration.
Muscles: Full body, shoulders, arms, waist, legs.
Joints: All.
Qi Flow: From the lower elixir field, it spirals to the shoulders, arms, and fingers as the arms are extended and stale essence is pulled out. Fresh essence is pulled in as one reforms the ball. It enters the body and is guided to where needed most.
Spiritual-Emotional: Centering yourself, then joyfully expanding your energy and consciousness outward.
Instructions: 1. Feet shoulder-width apart, knees slightly bent, you are holding a ball with your right hand under and left hand on top. Guide stale essence to your hands. 2. Turn your waist to the right and extend your right hand outward to eye level as you feel the stale essence pulling out. Hold momentarily to feel the fresh essence being pulled in. 3. Simultaneously, your left palm tucks under your left armpit extending to left; knees straighten slightly. The same pulling out and in is occurring in this hand.

4. Knees sink as you reform a ball of *qi* with your right hand on top and left hand under.
5. Turn your waist to the left and extend your left hand outward to eye level as your right palm tucks under your right armpit extending to right; knees straighten slightly. Essence is exchanged.

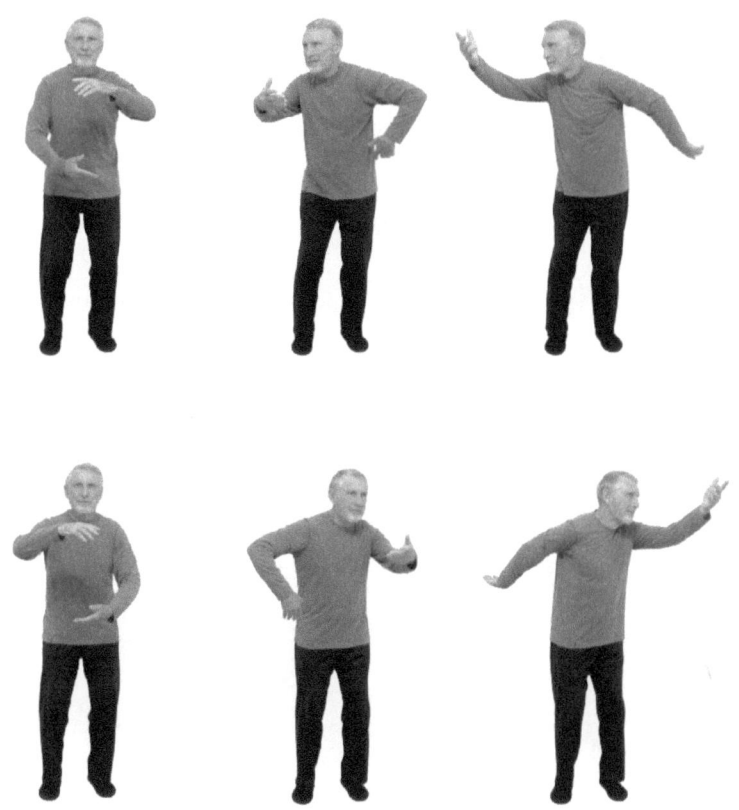

Ask Yourself

Are you smiling?

Are you relaxing?

Is the process of "guiding and pulling, pulling and guiding" making sense to you?

Chapter Five

Movements 12 through 22

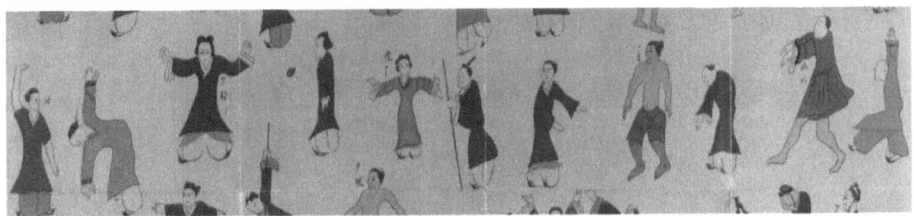

Fig. 5: The second row of *Daoyintu*.

This is the second row of movements as read from right to left. Seven of the eleven figures in this row are generally discernable in the original manuscript, however, #16, 18, and 22 are incomplete.

Daoyintu #13, 15, 20, and 22 treat specific ailments. There are stretches and balancing (#12, 13, 17, 21), meditation and breathing (#19), releasing (#12), and an animal movement (#20). After slow warmup, #12, 15, and 20 can be done forcefully to expel stale essence.

12. Giant Step (Y)

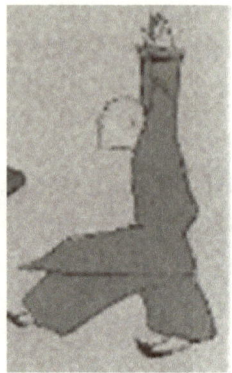

Actions: Stretching, balance, release of muscles, and emotional burden.
Muscles: Full body.
Joints: All.
Qi Flow: Rising to fingertips and simultaneously descending to the front leg and out the sole of that foot (through the *Yongquan* point), then rising back to the lower elixir field.
Spiritual-Emotional: Release (see Ch. 10 for the "Boulder Breath" story).
Instructions: 　1.　Feet shoulder-width apart. 　2.　Raise arms and take a long step forward with your left foot. 　3.　Bring your arms forward and down in a slow chopping motion that expels stale essence. Feel fresh essence pulled in through your fingers. 　4.　Sit back and turn your left foot outward 45 degrees. 　5.　Raise your arms again and step forward with your right foot, bringing your arms forward and down in a slow chopping motion that expels stale essence. 　6.　Turn 90 degrees to your left and pivot your feet to the left.

7. Repeat with left and right foot as above.
8. Perform these movements in each of the four cardinal directions.
9. After warmup, can be performed with comfortable force and speed.

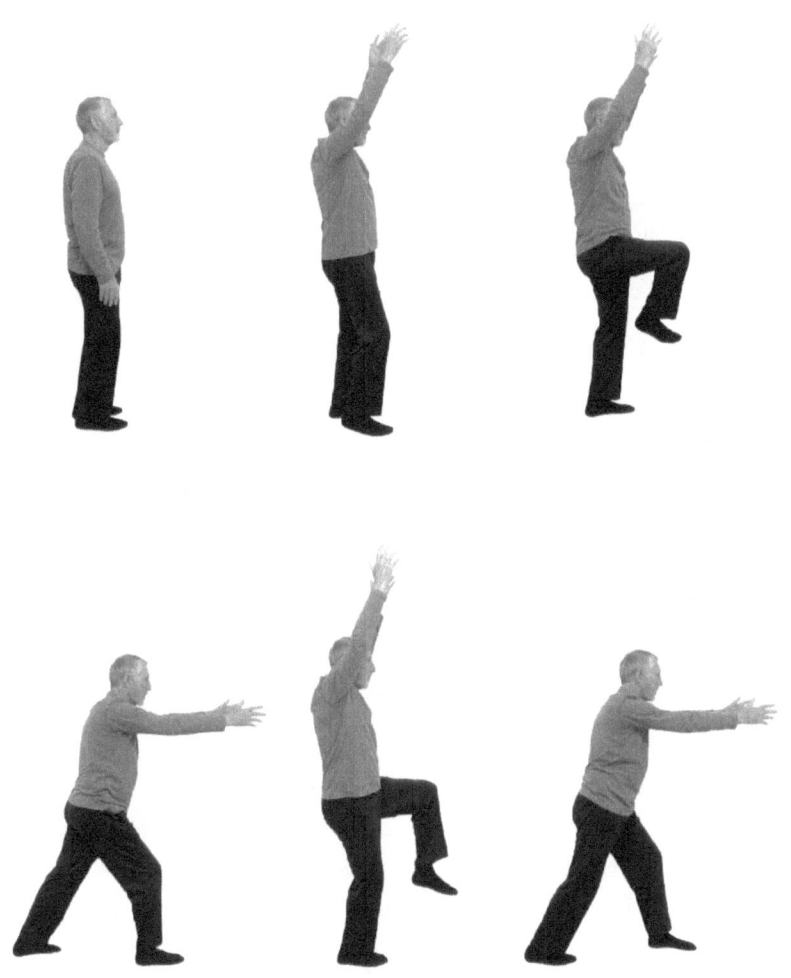

13. Slowly Extending Limbs (A)[1]

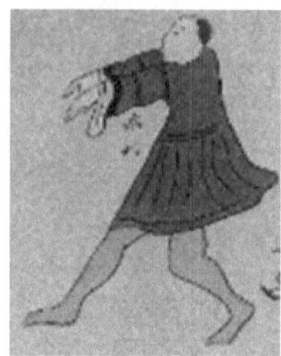

Actions: Stretching, balance, release, coordination.
Muscles: Rib cage, shoulders, intercostals, back, legs.
Joints: Ankles, knees, hips, shoulders.
Qi Flow: Rising through torso to shoulders and arms, also into extended leg.
Spiritual-Emotional: centering, release, confidence holding yourself steady, balance.
Instructions: 1. Feet shoulder-width apart. Focus on a point in the distance. 2. Extend your arms slowly, parallel to each other, in front, lifting your rib cage. 3. Lift and extend your left leg about 45 degrees and straighten your knee slowly, expelling stale essence. 4. Balance on your right leg for as long as comfortable while pulling in fresh essence. You can also keep your foot on the ground. 5. Stand on your left leg with both arms and right leg extended.

---

[1] Another translation is "For Pain in the Ribs," but this is not supported by Donald Harper (2009, 311n4).

Movements 12 through 22 / 53

6. An alternate method is to place the heel on the floor instead of lifting the leg.

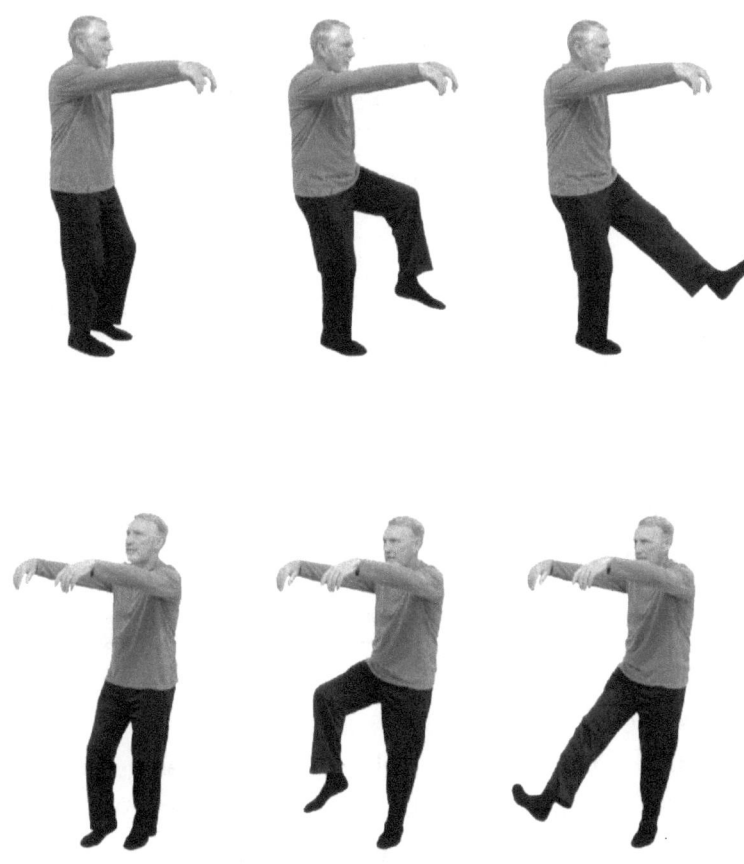

14. Gather Qi from Front and Back (A)

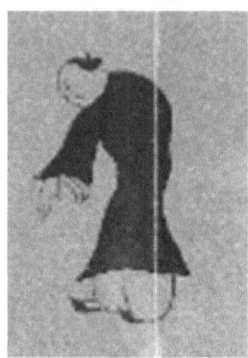

Actions: Gathering *qi*, stretching, loosening upper body and spine.
Muscles: Back, shoulders.
Joints: Shoulders, elbows, wrists, spine.
Qi Flow: Rising from the lower elixir field to shoulders, arms, and fingertips, sinking back to the elixir field, while more *qi* is gathered from the front and back.
Spiritual-Emotional: Energizing, gathering, nurturing.
Instructions: 1. Feet shoulder-width apart. 2. Circle your arms from behind your back and lean forward about 45 degrees to hold a large ball in front of your chest. 3. Turn your palms upward and bring them to your Lower Elixir Field as you straighten your back.

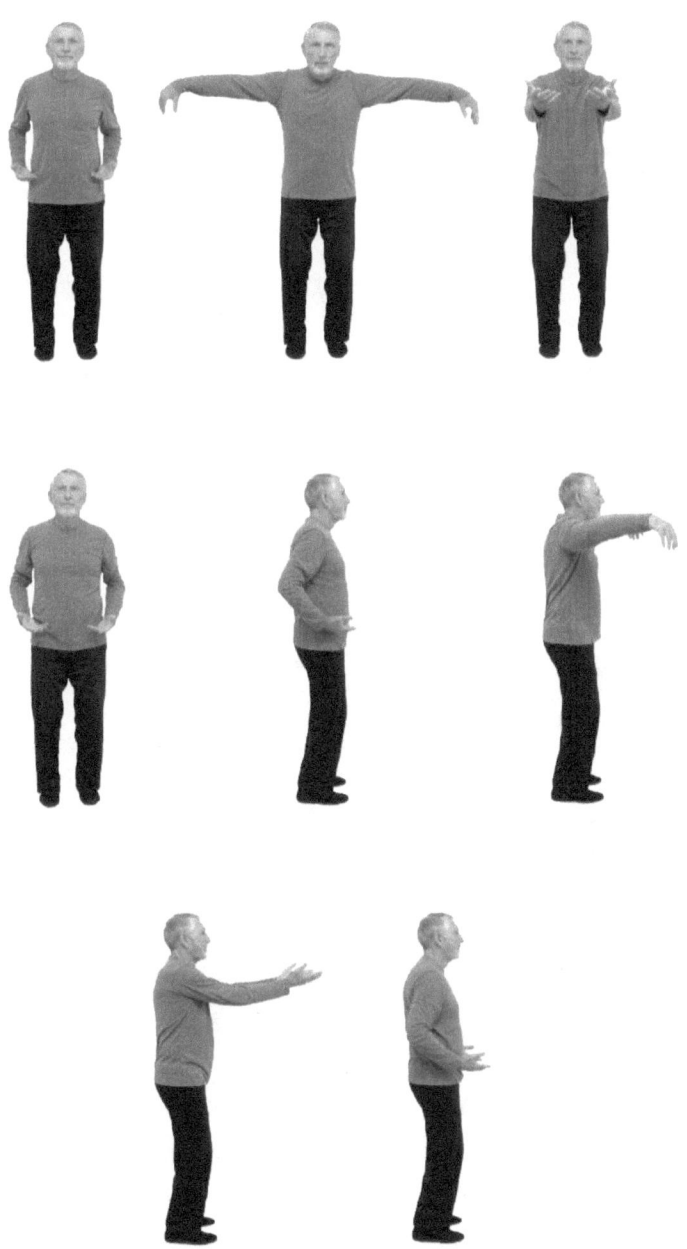

15. Bouncing the Elixir Field (A)

Pulling Inguinal Swelling (H)

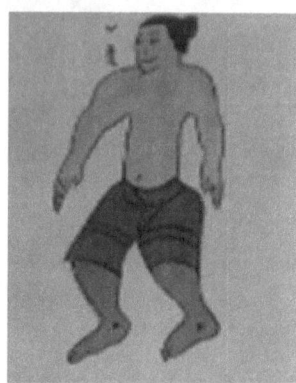

Actions: Breathing, bouncing, vibration releases fascia, induces lymphatic drainage, organ massage, stimulating the triple heater.
Muscles: Legs, abdominals, back, shoulders, and arms.
Joints: Knees, ankles, hips, shoulders.
Qi Flow: Spinning *qi* in the lower elixir field, it rises and falls as one bounces. Stale *qi* is emitted through the Yongquan point on the soles of feet and the fingertips.
Spiritual-Emotional: Release, shaking off your troubles, joy of bouncing.

Instructions:
  1. Feet shoulder-width apart.
  2. Use focused intention to spin the lower elixir field internally.
  3. Start an up and down bouncing movement and coordinate the lower elixir field spin with your bounces.
  4. Exhale as you drop and inhale as you rise.
  5. Try each of the healing sounds: "shoe," "chway," and "hoo."

6. Do the bounces slowly to feel pulling out and in through the soles of your feet and fingers. Optionally do them faster and more forcefully, as long as you can do them without discomfort.

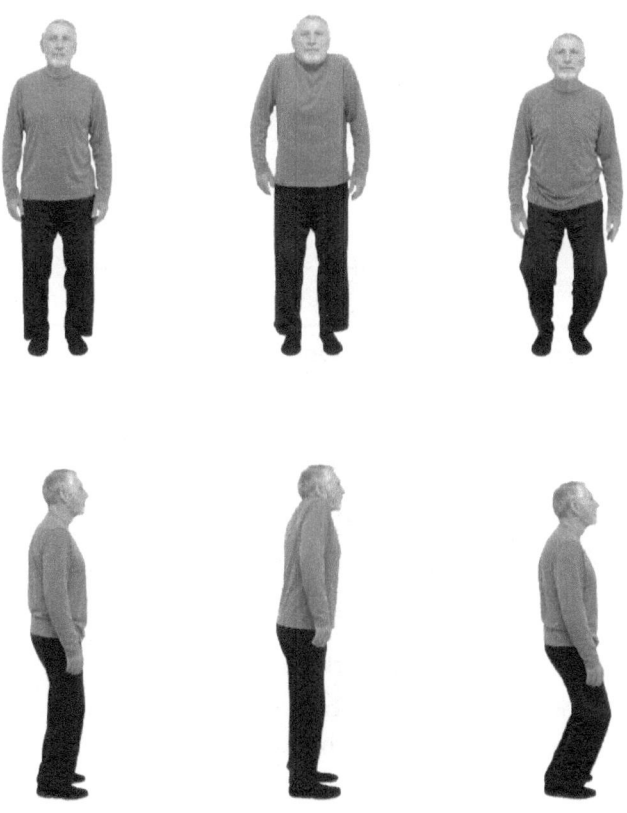

16. Swinging Arms (A)

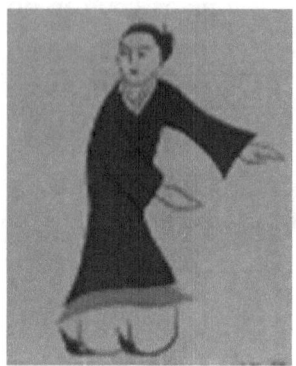

Actions: Stretching, twisting, organ massage.
Muscles: Back, abdominals, shoulders, arms, neck.
Joints: Back, hips, shoulders, neck.
Qi Flow: Ascending with arm raise, descending back to the lower elixir field and down to the feet as the arms drop.
Spiritual-Emotional: Reaching for a star (aspirational goal), release.
Instructions: 1. Feet shoulder-width apart, with torso straight. 2. Standing straight, swing both arms up and to one side, turning your head to watch your hands rise. 3. Let your arms fall, bending your knees slightly as you do. 4. Swing your arms to the other side, again following the movement with your eyes.

Movements 12 through 22 / 59

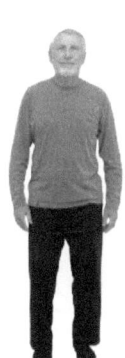 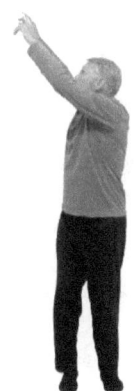 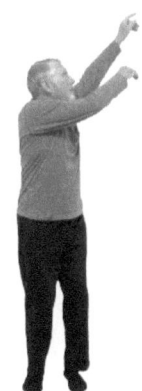

17. Pole Rock (A)

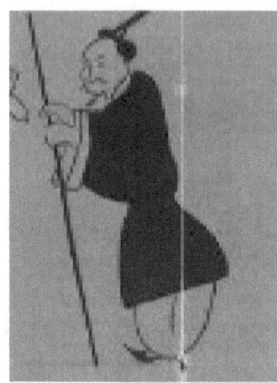

Actions: Stretching, balancing, loosening the sacrum.
Muscles: Legs, calves, back, shoulders.
Joints: Ankles, knees, hips.
Qi Flow: Bending forward builds *qi* "pressure," released as one straightens. Feel the *qi* rising from the feet to the perineum, then on to the sacrum, up the spine to the *Baihui* (Hundred Meeting) point at the top of the head. From there, *qi* sinks back to the lower elixir field and feet. Use the end of the pole to stimulate the *Laogong* (Labor Palace) points in the center of the palms, then try moving *qi* through the pole.
Spiritual-Emotional: aligning self, depending/trusting (on the support of the pole or wall), being balanced, "leaning in."
Instructions: 1. Feet shoulder-width apart. 2. Use a long pole, or place your palms against a wall for stability. 3. Lean into the pole or wall, while inhaling, and shift your weight onto your heels. 4. Straighten up and raise your heels. Feel stale essence being released through your feet, *Bai Hui*, and hands/*Lao Gong* points as you exhale.

5. Fresh essence flows in as your feet reconnect with the ground.

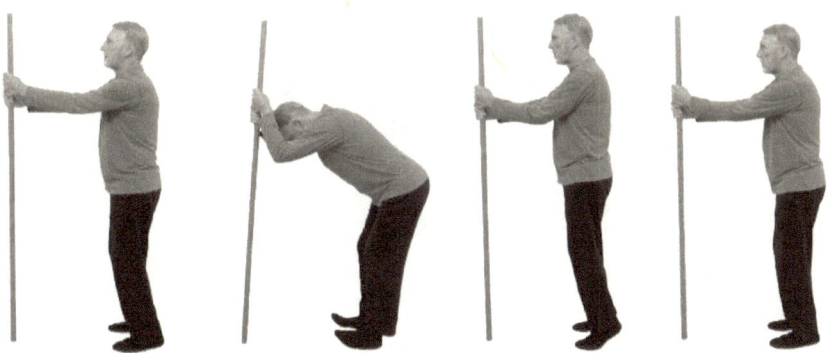

18. Inside the Abdomen (H)

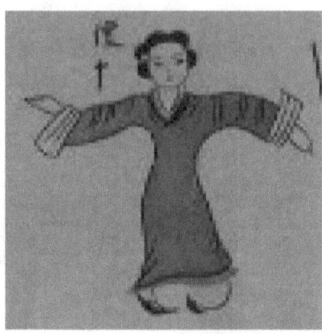

Actions: *Qi* gathering, visualization and manipulation, exercise for shoulders, upper body coordination.
Muscles: Shoulders, arms, upper back.
Joints: Shoulders, wrists, neck.
Qi Flow: Rising from feet and the lower elixir field to shoulders, out the shoulder and into the upraised hand. It also moves across the shoulders and through the arms to the other hand, then it sinks back to the lower elixir field.
Spiritual-Emotional: Flowing, drifting *qi*, imagination.
Instructions: 1. Feet shoulder-width apart or wider. 2. Arms extended to the sides with left palm facing up and right palm facing down. Imagine or feel a ball of *qi* in your left hand. 3. As you raise your left arm and hand, your right arm and hand descends slowly. 4. Imagine/feel the ball of *qi* roll down your left arm, across your shoulders to your right hand as you rotate your right wrist to turn your palm upward and catch the ball. 5. Then lift your right arm up while allowing your left arm and hand (now turned palm down) to descend.

6. Imagine/feel the ball of *qi* roll down your right arm, across your shoulders to your left hand, where you catch it.
7. Now imagine your *qi* sinking to the lower elixir field.

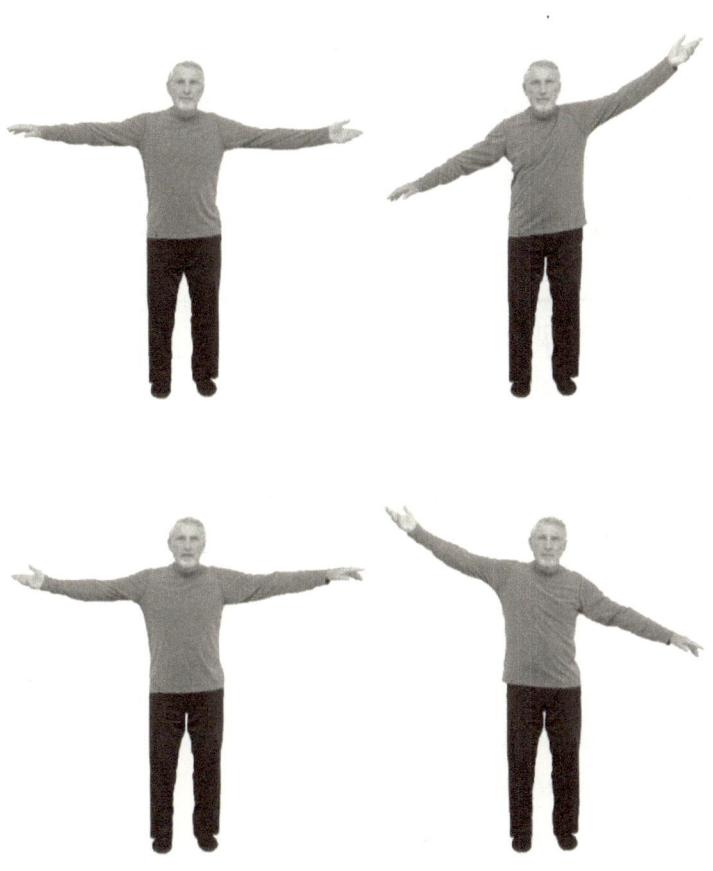

64 / Chapter Five

19. Centered Breathing (A)

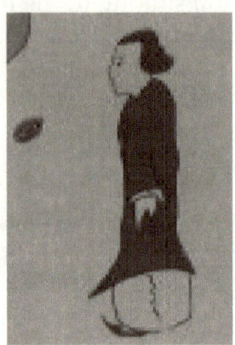

Actions: Breathing practice, meditation.
Muscles: Chest, diaphragm.
Joints: Ribs.
Qi Flow: Rising from feet to top of head and down or from the lower elixir field up the spine and back down.
Spiritual-Emotional: Savoring your breath, relaxation, meditation, centering.
Instructions: 1. Feet shoulder-width apart. 2. Arms by sides and entire body relaxed. 3. Inhale for 5 seconds, exhale for 5 seconds. Bend knees as you exhale. Use healing sounds, if desired. 4. Inhale for 10 seconds, and straighten knees, exhale for 10 seconds, bend knees. 5. Inhale for 15 seconds, exhale for 15; inhale for 20, exhale for 20, continuing to increase duration as you are able.

Movements 12 through 22 / 65

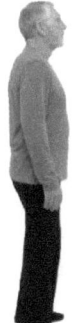 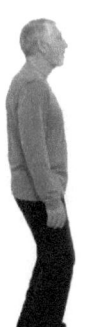 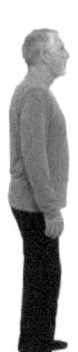

20. Bear Drops (A)

Pulling Deafness[2] (H)

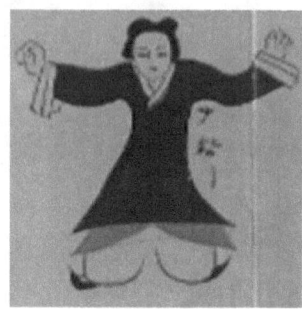

Actions: Stretching, bouncing, release, massaging internal organs, hearing exercise.
Muscles: Arms, shoulders, legs.
Joints: All.
Qi Flow: Rising up the back to shoulders, arms, fingertips, and head, then sinking back to the lower elixir field and the soles of the feet.
Spiritual-Emotional: Connection with bear, shaking off hesitancy, releasing fear.
Instructions: 1. Feet shoulder-width apart or wider.   2. On the first set, reach up slowly with arms partially spread, imagine grasping a branch with your "paws."   3. Drop your hips while exhaling explosively. Try "shoe," "shway," and "hoo."   4. Your stale essence is pulled out.

---

[2] In the system of the five phases, the bear is associated with the ears, the phase water, the color black or indigo, and the kidneys (see App 2).

5. As you rise, fresh essence is pulled in.
6. On the second set reach up and cross your wrists, then drop hips, while exhaling explosively.
7. Pause, concentrate on your ears and try to hear sounds in the distance.

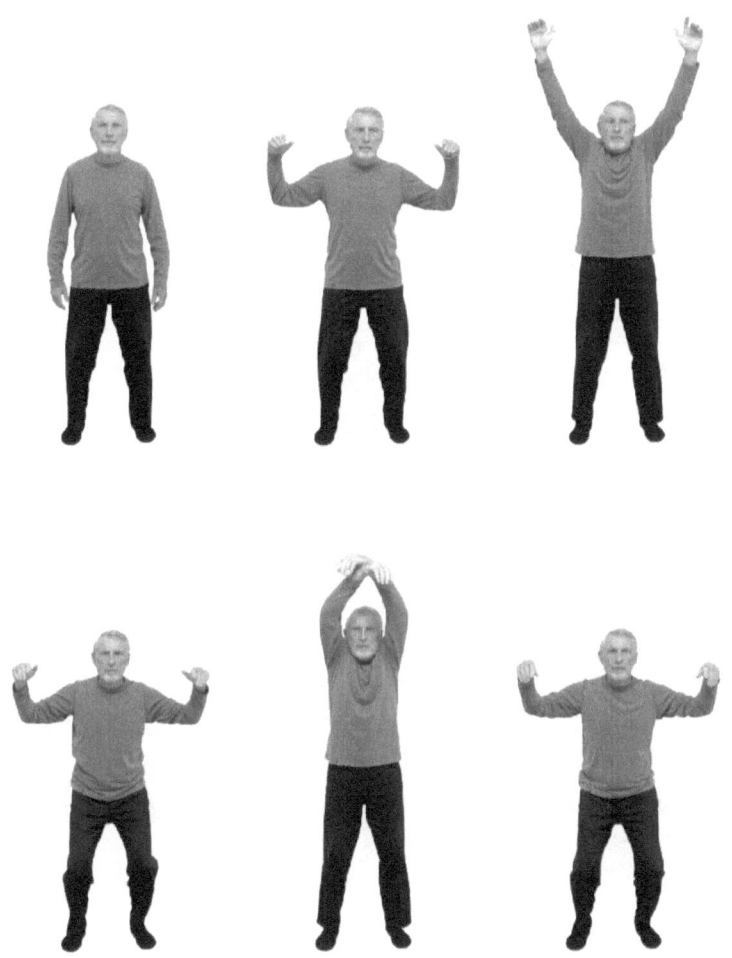

21. Picking Up an Apple (Y)

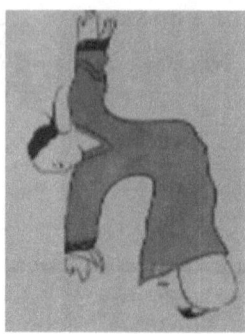

Actions: Stretching, flexibility.
Muscles: Back, shoulders, arms, legs.
Joints: Hips, shoulders, neck.
Qi Flow: Rising from the lower elixir field through the back to the arms and hands, exchanging *qi* with the earth, then sinking back to the lower elixir field as one straightens up.
Spiritual-Emotional: Exchanging *qi* with earth.
Instructions: 　1.　Feet shoulder-width apart. 　2.　Bend forward as if picking up an apple with your right hand, while extending the left arm upwards (imagine you are extending your reach into the earth to pull out stale essence and then pull fresh essence in). 　3.　Keep your back as still as you can while you move your shoulders. 　4.　Reach to the earth with your left hand while extending the right arm upwards. 　5.　Alternate arms as you remain bent over.

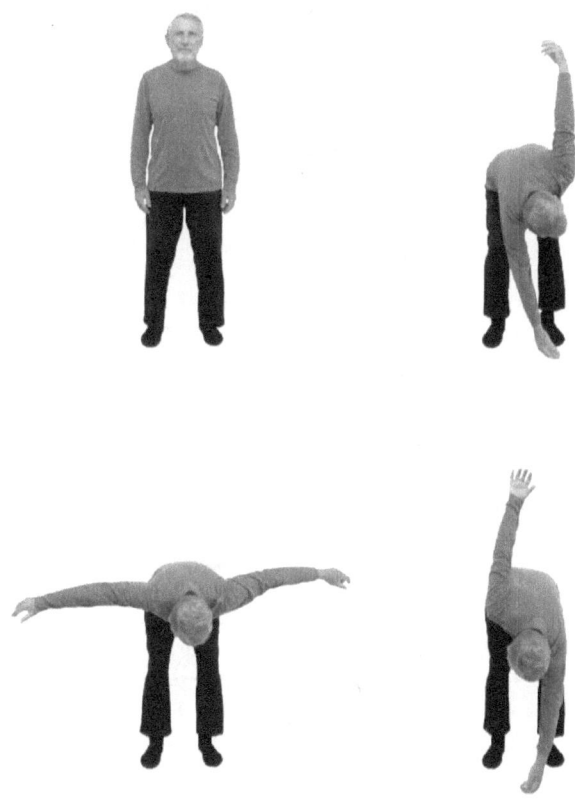

22. Connection with heaven (A)

Feverishness, Possibly of the Heart. (H)

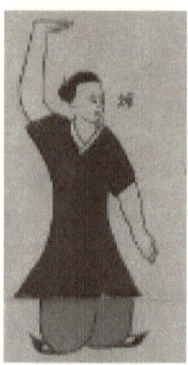

Actions: stretching, linking with "heavenly" *qi*. Compliments #21.
Muscles: shoulders, arms, neck.
Joints: shoulder, elbow, wrist, neck.
Qi Flow: Rising from the lower elixir field to the palms (*Laogong* point) and the top of the head (*Baihui*), then sinking down again to the lower elixir field.
Spiritual-Emotional: opening upper body to heaven; glaring eyes as the head turns, restores confidence.
Instructions: 1. Feet shoulder-width apart. 2. Lift your right arm overhead, turning the palm up with your fingers pointing left. 3. Turn your head and look left, exhaling "shoe" as you do. Feel stale essence being pulled out and replaced by fresh essence. 4. Bring your right arm down by your side as you look straight forward.

5. Lift your left arm overhead, turning the palm up with your fingers pointing right.
6. Turn your head and look right, exhaling "shoe" as you do.
7. Bring your left arm down and look straight forward. Repeat.

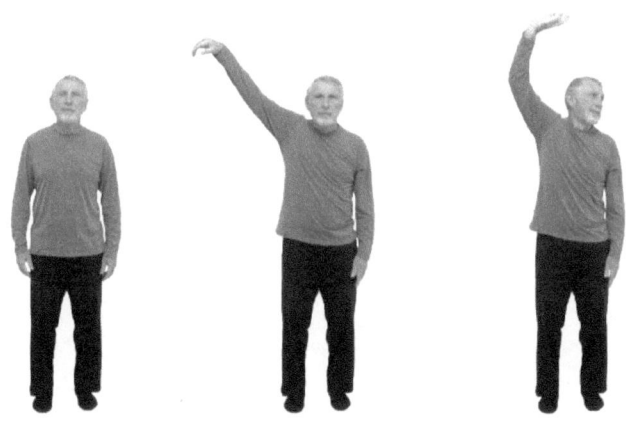

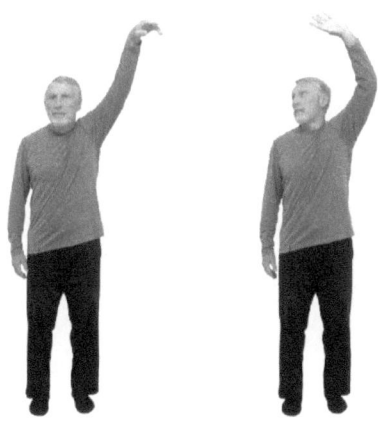

Chapter Six

Movements 23 through 33

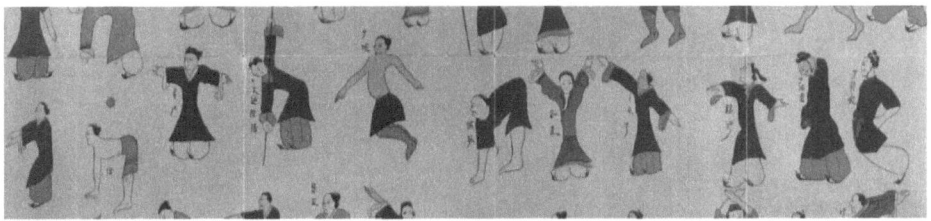

Fig. 6: The third row of *Daoyintu*.

This is the third row of movements as read from right to left. Ten of the pictures are discernable in the original manuscript, and only #29 is incomplete. Therefore, this row is the most representative of the work of the original artist or artists.

These movements are also varied in their application. Specific ailments are addressed in #23 and 24. In addition, we consider #24 to be meditational (see also chapter 8). Six of the images—#25, 26, 27, 29, 32 and 33—depict releasing movements. The underlying theme of this row seems to be animals. If you include dragons, #25, 27, 28, 32, and 33 are all about animal movements. Crane Call, #25, indicates that some sort of bird sound was made. Figures #23, 25, 26, 30 31, and 33 are clear examples of pulling stale essence, and #33 can be done forcefully, if desired.

23. Hip and Knee Bend (A)

Pulling Knee Pain (H)

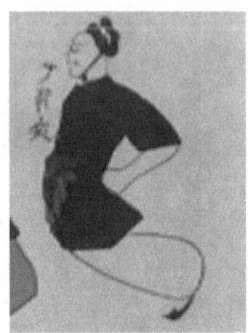

Actions: Stretch front of body, organ massage, opening sacrum.
Muscles: Shoulders, back, chest, gluteus, legs, especially knee muscles.
Joints: Hips, knees, spine.
Qi Flow: Rising from the lower elixir field to the *Mingmen* point and the kidneys, and on from there to the heart and lungs.
Spiritual-Emotional: Alleviating fear, comforting.
Instructions: 1. Stand with feet shoulder-width apart, or may be done kneeling. 2. Place fists on kidneys, then massage your kidneys as you bend backwards from your waist, without straining. 3. Guide and pull stale essence, including pain, to be exhaled with any sound you wish to make. 4. Bend forwards from your waist, again without straining and inhale. 5. Repeat by bending back and forth deliberately. 6. You can also place fists on your sacrum as you bend.

Movements 23 through 33 / 75

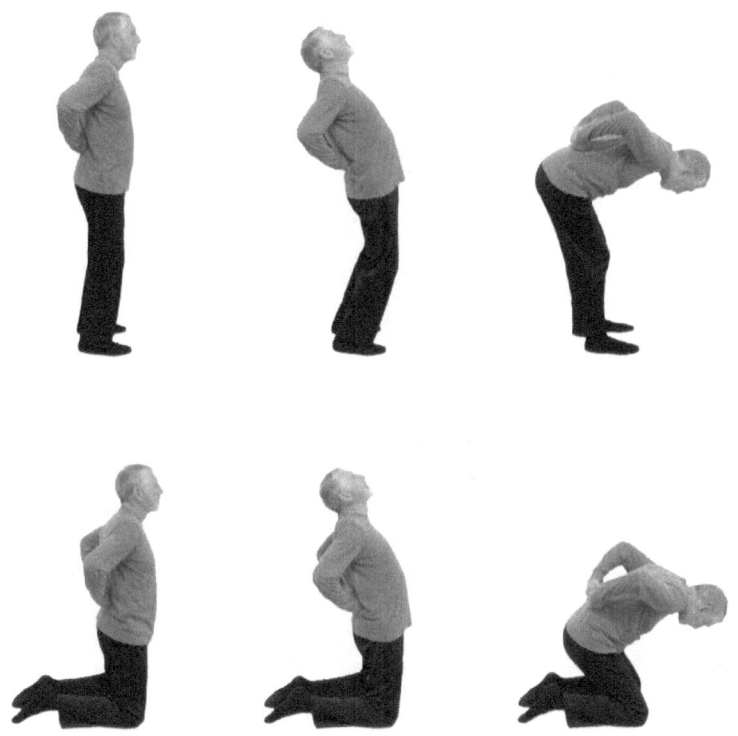

24. Carry Money (Y)

Pulling Upper Side Accumulation (H)

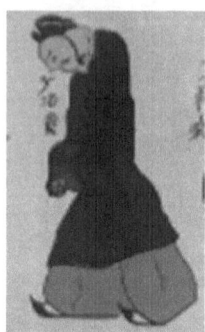

Actions: Breathing, meditation, mindful walking, balance, relieving an energy, emotional, or mental blockage.
Muscles: Legs, neck.
Joints: Ankles, knees, cervical.
Qi Flow: Sinking from the top of the head all the way down to each foot to make full contact with the earth. Take in fresh *qi* through the foot upon inhalation.
Spiritual-Emotional: Internal immersion. Relaxation, concentration, being closed to the world, you are in the sanctuary of yourself.

Instructions:
  1. Interlace fingers with palms facing up; bring your chin to your chest and relax your shoulders. Close your eyes.
  2. Take a small step forward, placing your heel first, then exhaling as you shift weight gradually to your whole foot (your breathing controls your steps).
  3. Repeat with your other foot.
  4. You can walk in a straight line, a curve, or a circle, or other pattern.

5. You can also walk backwards, placing your toes down first and then shifting your weight to your whole foot.

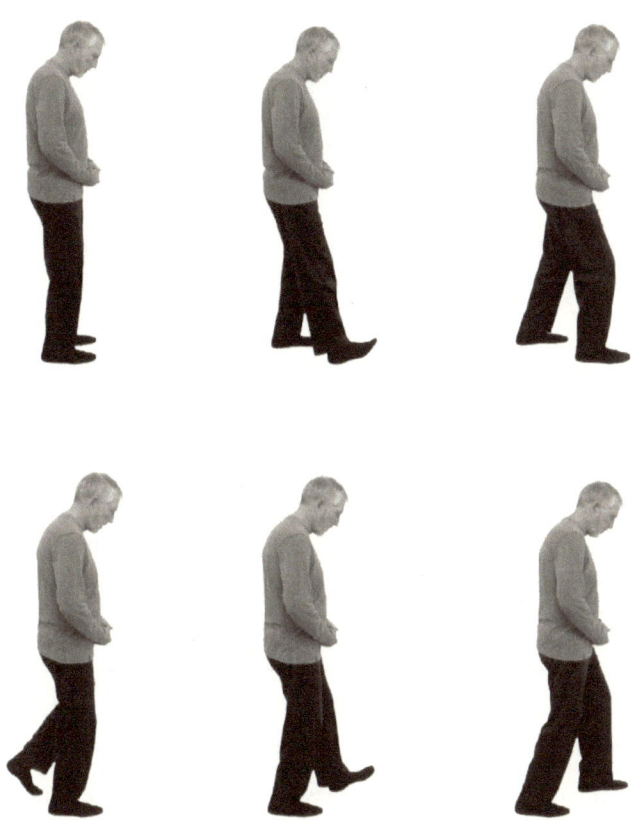

25. Crane Call (K)

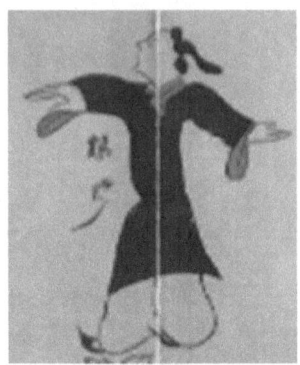

Actions: Stretching, relaxation, flexibility.
Muscles: Back, arms, legs.
Joints: Ankles, knees, wrists, shoulders, elbows.
Qi Flow: Rising from the lower elixir field to shoulders, arms, and hands, sinking back to the lower elixir field and down through the legs.
Spiritual-Emotional: Imagination, flying with the Crane.
Instructions: 1. Feet shoulder-width apart, palms down and wrists flexible. 2. Bring right arm (wing) forward in front of you and the other arm back, behind you. 3. Rise up and inhale, as your "wings" come up while guiding stale essence to your extremities. 4. As your "wings" come down, exhale stale essence and sink, bending your knees. 5. Inhale fresh essence as you bring your left "wing" up and your right "wing" back, behind you and repeat. 6. In keeping with the movement's name, you can make a crane noise if you wish.

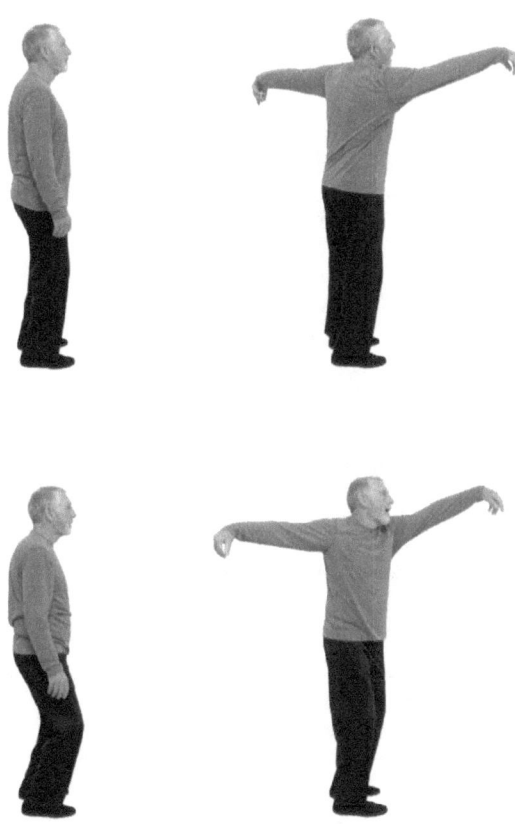

26. Slanted Flying (A)

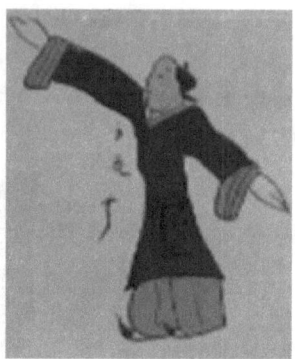

Actions: Stretching, opening, concentration.
Muscles: Neck, shoulders, arms, waist.
Joints: Shoulders, elbows, wrists, neck.
Qi Flow: Rising along the back from the lower elixir field, across the shoulders to the fingertips and back to the lower elixir field.
Spiritual-Emotional: Opening, release, lightness of spirit.
Instructions: 1. Feet shoulder-width apart. 2. Start with your right palm facing up, under your left palm, which is facing down. in front of the lower elixir field. 3. Extend arms with right hand 45 degrees above horizontal and left hand 45 degree below horizontal. Pull stale essence from your fingertips. 4. Turn head and shoulders to focus your eyes on the right hand. 5. Return your hands to the lower elixir field with the right hand on top and the left hand underneath. 6. Extend your left arm 45 degrees up and right hand 45 degrees down. Pull stale essence.

Movements 23 through 33 / 81

> 7. Turn head and shoulders to focus your eyes on the left hand.

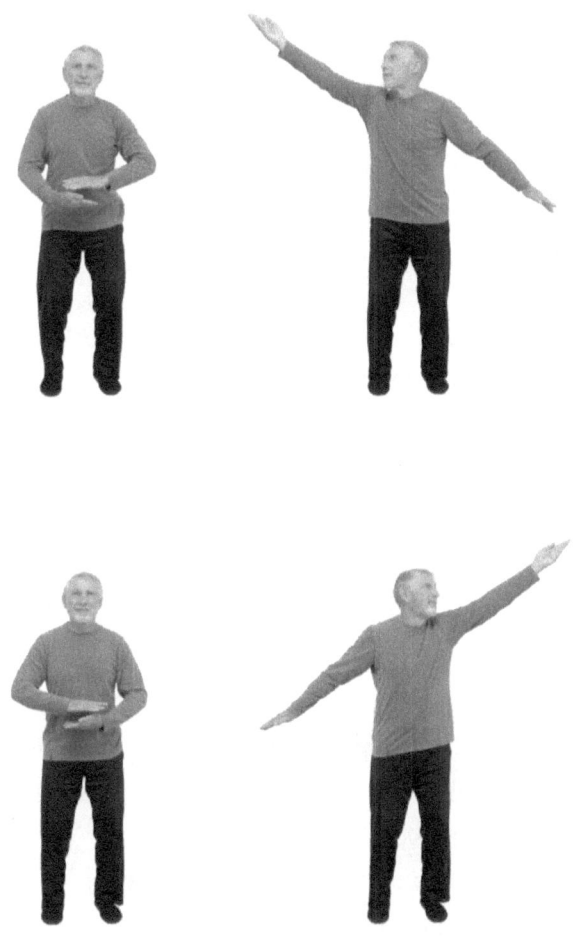

27. Dragon Ascending (H)

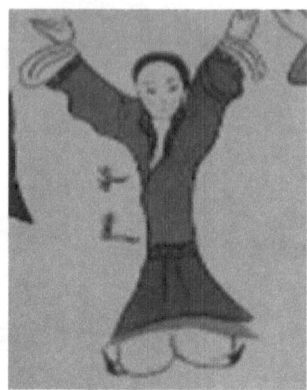

Actions: Stretching, opening, releasing.
Muscles: All.
Joints: All, entire body.
Qi Flow: Rising through your body to the fingertips and back down.
Spiritual-Emotional: Emergence, unbridled release of yang energy, imaginative connection with dragon.
Instructions: 1. Take a short step to your left, feet shoulder-width apart or wider, palms down. 2. Squat and cross your wrists. 3. Straighten your legs, bringing your wrists up to your midline. 4. Separate your wrists and spread your arms open above your head. 5. Bring your wrists towards each other and down, crossing them as you reach your midline. 6. As you squat, uncross your wrists, spreading your arms wide. 7. Cross your wrists as before and rise again.

Movements 23 through 33 / 83

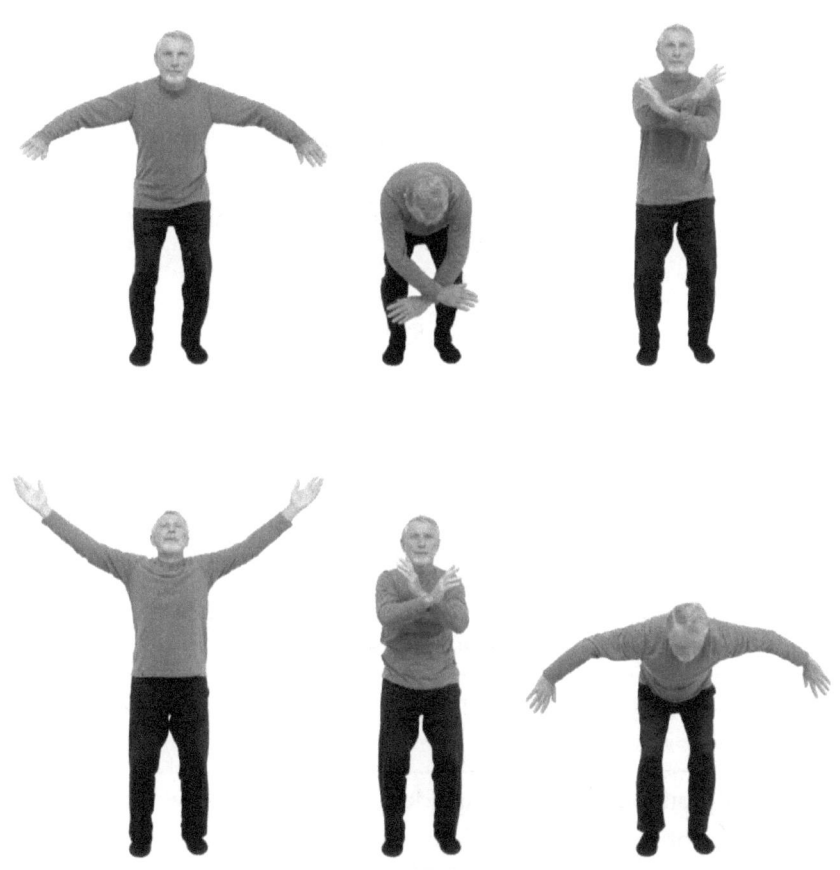

28. Tiger Backs into Cave (Y)

Bending Down for Reversal. (H)

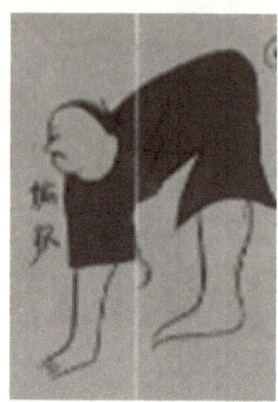

What it does – Restores natural flow of *qi*.
Muscles: All.
Joints: Ankles, knees, hips, shoulders, neck.
Qi Flow: Rising through the body, up the back to arms and hands, then again to the lower elixir field.
Spiritual-Emotional: Rebalancing, identifying with the tiger, warily taking measure of a problem from a protected position.
Instructions: 1. Feet shoulder-width apart, or wider, palms down. 2. Bend over, with your palms (paws) near or touching the ground. 3. Draw in your chin slightly and lift head to look forward This may not be easy for some practitioners, so do this movement very cautiously. Your eyes should glare. 4. Move your legs and arms to walk, in very short steps, backwards as though entering a cave hindquarter first.

5. Try to do this for a count of ten, then slowly straighten up. As you exhale, try "shoe," "chway," and "hoo" sounds.
6. Pause to feel your energy and repeat.

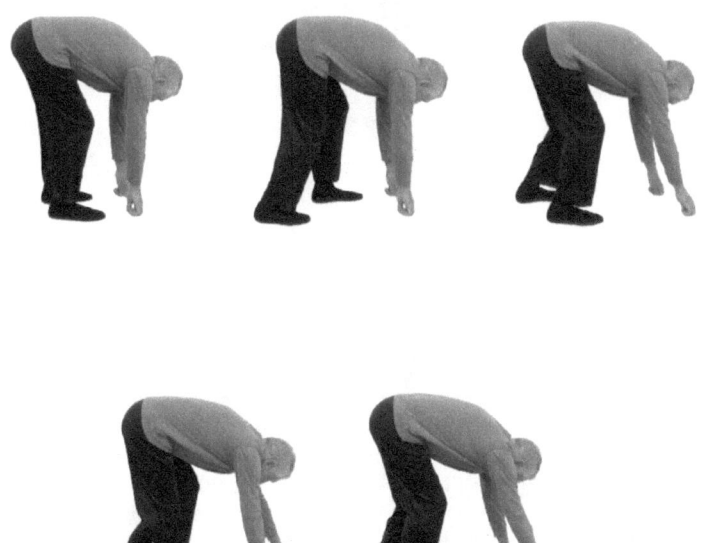

29. Looking Back (A)

Pulling the Nape (H)

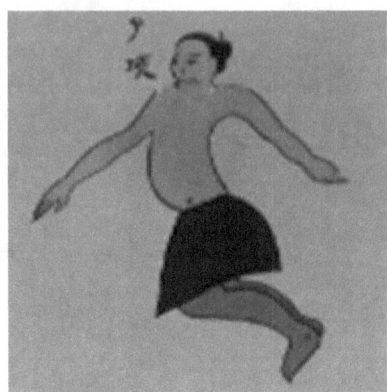

Actions: Stretching the neck, loosening, flexibility.
Muscles: Legs, hips, waist, chest, shoulders, neck.
Joints: Neck, knees, hips, back, shoulders.
Qi Flow: Rising from the soles of the feet up the legs to torso, arms, hands, and head.
Spiritual-Emotional: Retrospection in motion, focus, relaxation.

1. Feet shoulder-width apart, or closer, depending on your balance.
2. Raise arms with both palms facing upwards; right hand in front of you and left one in back.
3. Turn to look back at your left hand.
4. Return arms to your sides, while sinking (bending your knees) at the same time.
5. As you raise your arms, with left hand in front, rise by straightening your legs as you look back at your right hand.

Movements 23 through 33 / 87

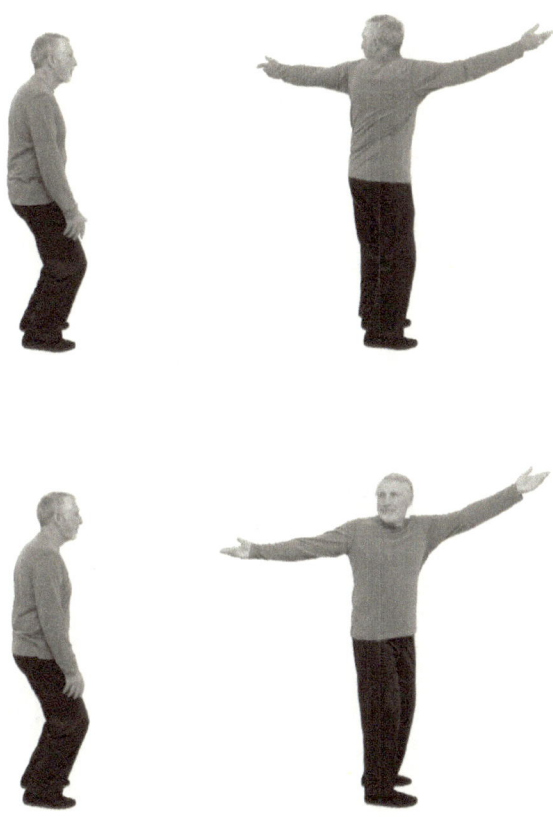

30. Penetrating *Yin* and *Yang* with a Pole (H)

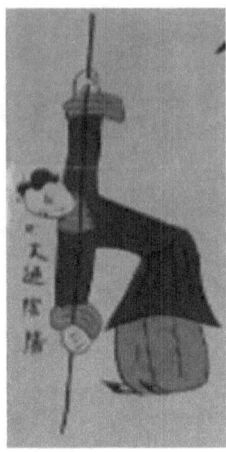

Actions: Stretching, loosening, enhancing flexibility, strengthening.
Muscles: Back, shoulders, arms.
Joints: Hips, spine, shoulders.
Qi Flow: The pole is a tool for connecting yin and yang. Qi rises from the lower elixir field up the back to shoulders and arms. Stale essence can be discharged through the pole, and fresh essence received through the pole via the *Laogong* points.
Spiritual-Emotional: Balancing energies of heaven and earth.
Instructions (also possible without a pole):   1. Feet shoulder-width apart, or wider. This is a physically challenging movement, be cautious.   2. Hold a pole horizontally; both hands grasp the pole with knuckles facing up (width between hands can be from about 1 foot to 4 feet).   3. Bend at the waist while extending both arms, turning so that your right hand (while grasping the pole) is nearest to the earth.

The pole should be as vertical as possible. Relax and feel the exchange of qi.

4. Then turn to the other side so that your left hand is nearest to the earth.

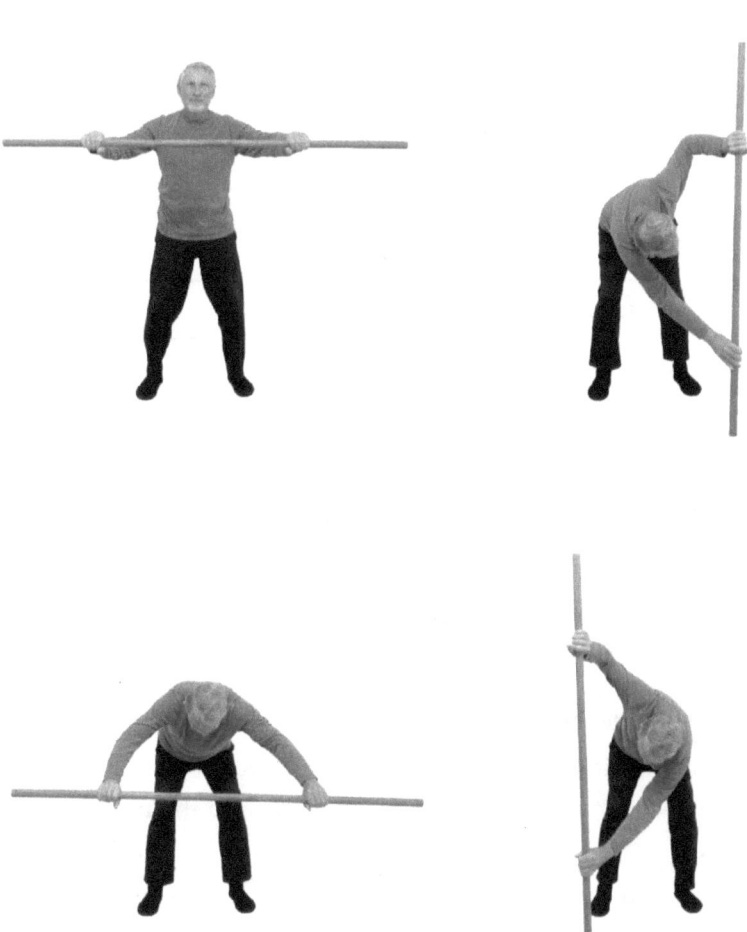

31. Swinging the Upper Arms (H)

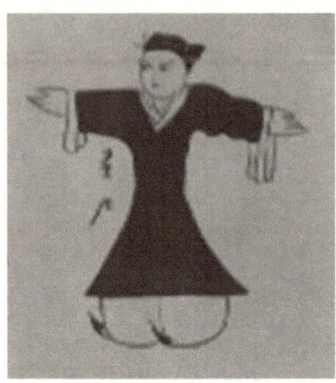

Actions: Stretching, loosening, balance.
Muscles: Shoulders, arms, lower back, legs.
Joints: Shoulders, scapulae, elbows, wrists, ankles.
Qi Flow: Rising from the lower elixir field, up the spine, out through the arms to the fingertips and back down to Yongquan points on the soles of the feet.
Spiritual-Emotional: Feeling lightness, soaring free, being above it all.
Instructions: <ol><li>Feet shoulder-width apart, or wider, with relaxed hands.</li><li>Bring arms in front, then bend slightly forward, while tucking hands under armpits and extending them to the back, palms up.</li><li>Guide and pull stale essence from your fingers as you look straight forward.</li><li>Lift both palms a bit higher (you will feel it in your shoulders) and at the same time rise up on your toes. Balance there for as long as you are comfortable while pulling in fresh essence.</li><li>Relax, let your hands fall to your sides and repeat when ready.</li></ol>

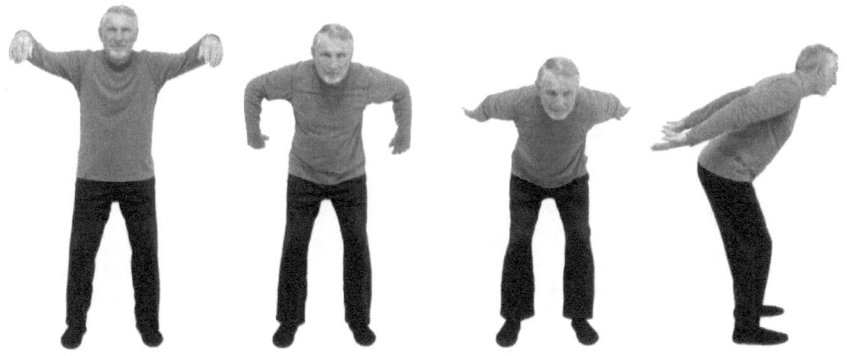

32. Bird Stretch (Y)

Chicken stretch (H)

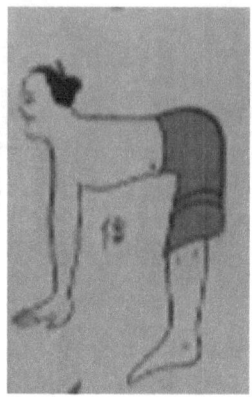

Actions: Stretching, releasing muscles, and fascia. Clearing.
Muscles: Back, shoulders, arms.
Joints: Hips, back, shoulders, elbows, wrists, fingers.
Qi Flow: rising from torso into raised hands, expels to earth and out the fingers, then descends back to the lower elixir field and earth.
Spiritual-Emotional: cleansing, as one emulates a bird washing its wings and flicking away cares like water.
Instructions: 1. Feet shoulder-width apart, or wider. Spread your arms (wings). 2. Bend from the waist, bringing your hands forward, then down toward the earth. Exhale. 3. As you continue to exhale, extend your arms to the sides, while still bending over, and flutter your wrists and hands 4. Inhale as you straighten and repeat.

Movements 23 through 33 / 93

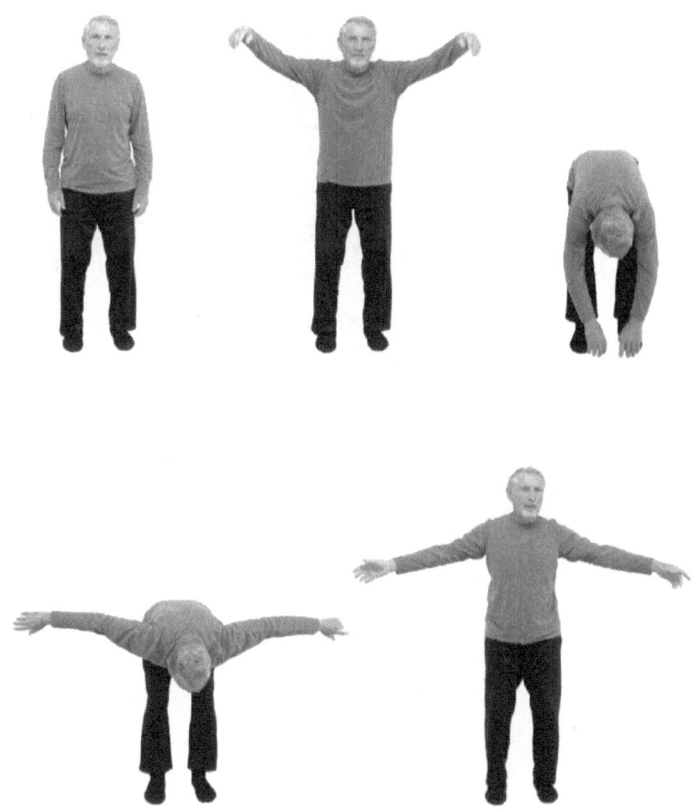

33. Big Bird (Y)

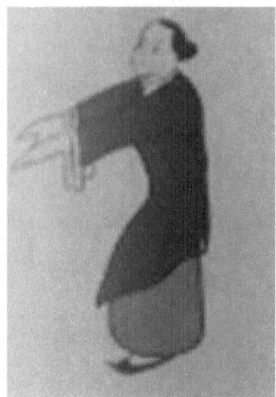

Actions: stretching, waist flexibility, release anger and stale essence.
Muscles: shoulders, upper back, waist.
Joints: shoulder, elbow.
Qi Flow: rising from the lower elixir field up spine to shoulders and down arms to fingertips. Stale essence is expelled through your fingers.
Spiritual-Emotional: quick release, cleansing.
Instructions: 1. Feet shoulder-width apart, or wider.   2. Fingers are straight, but relaxed.   3. Slowly and fully extend both arms to one side at a 45-dgree angle, guiding and pulling stale essence while exhaling. Your relaxed fingers may vibrate.   4. Retract both arms while pulling in fresh essence. Move your arms to the other side at a 45-degree angle and extend them again, while exhaling. Try sounds "shoe," "shway," and "hoo."   5. Take your time, to appreciate the guiding and pulling. Increase speed and forcefulness, doing multiple extensions as desired.

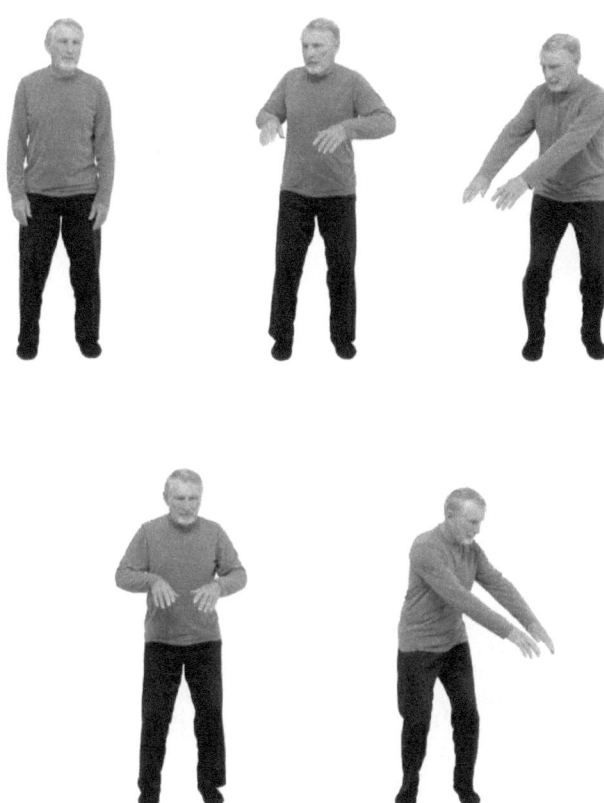

Chapter Seven

Movements 34 through 44

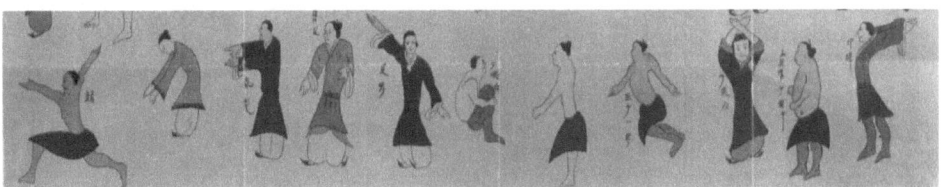

Figure 7: The bottom row of *Daoyintu*.

This is the fourth row of movements as read from right to left. Four of its eleven figures are incomplete in the original manuscript, that is, #38, 40, 43, and 44. This is arguably the most complex row of movements.

Movements #35 and 36 address overheated conditions, and #39 is for pain in the buttocks. Images #35, 40, 41, 42, and 44 are animal movements. The titles of #34 and 35 indicate noises are made "(Looking up and Shouting" and "Monkey Bawling").

Good examples of pulling stale essence are #34, 36, 37, 40, 41, and 43. After warmup, #34, 35, 36, and 38 can be done forcefully.

To the authors, #37, 42, and 43 seem to significantly enhance connection with, and accumulation of, *qi*. The final image, #44, could be the most challenging movement of them all. Perhaps performing it successfully validated a completed course of treatment.

34. Look Up and Shout (H)

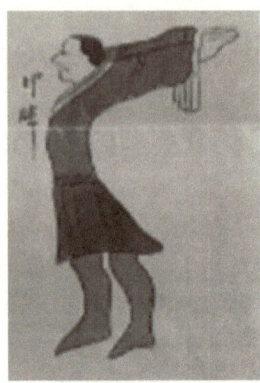

Actions: Stretching, releasing, clearing the lungs.
Muscles: Chest, pectorals, shoulders, arms, neck.
Joints: Shoulders, back, neck.
Qi Flow: Rising from the lower elixir field up the back to shoulders and out to the hands; then the *qi* descends down the body and returns to the lower elixir field.
Spiritual-Emotional: Release grief and anger.
Instructions: 1. Please note that #34 is anatomically impossible, as drawn, so the movements have been modified. 2. Feet shoulder-width apart, or wider. 3. Extend your arms in front of your body at shoulder height, palms together. 4. As you exhale, move your arms down by your sides and then lift them as high as you comfortably can behind your back. 5. Your palms are facing down. 6. As you bend your neck slowly back and look up, exhale; you may feel naturally compelled to shout, as stale essence is pulled out. A healing sound could also be voiced.

Movements 34 through 44 / 99

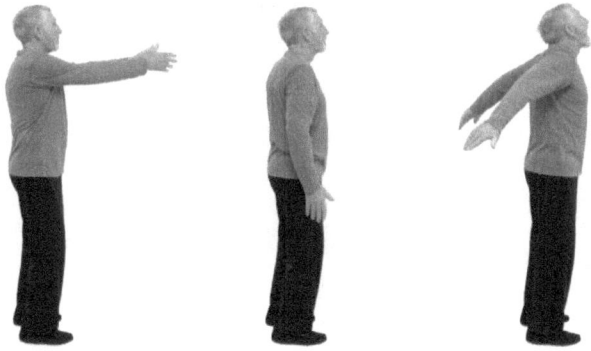

35. Monkey Bawling: To Pull Internal Heat (H)

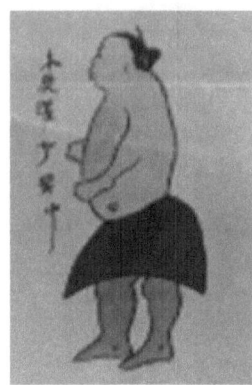

Actions: Releases internal heat from lower and middle *Jiao* by bouncing and sound vibration. The figure indicates abdominal expansion.
Muscles: Legs, gluteus, abdominals, chest.
Joints: Ankles, knees, elbows, shoulders.
Qi Flow: Rapid oscillation clears, excites, and amplifies the energy in the body.
Spiritual-Emotional: Releasing emotions, especially anger and frustration. Anger and heat are related.

Instructions:
    1. Feet shoulder-width apart, or wider.
    2. Make medium loose fists with loose arms.
    3. Bounce up and down, keeping feet flat on the ground.
    4. Make a sound as you exhale. Suggested sounds: "shoe" or "hoo-hoo," but experiment with any other sounds that come naturally.

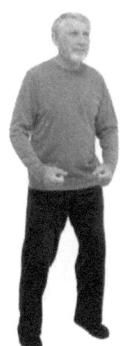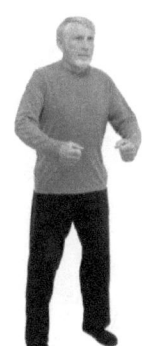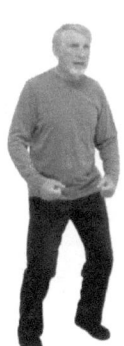

36. Pulling the Warm Ailment (H)

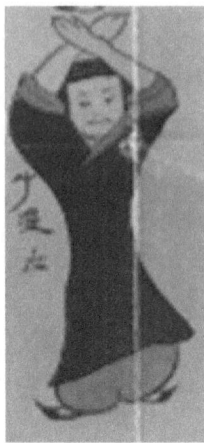

Actions: Releasing heat, stretching, opening, forcefully expelling air, emotions.
Muscles: Back, shoulders, arms.
Joints: Wrists, elbows, shoulders, spine.
Qi Flow: Guiding and pulling from the head and hands into the earth as you bend forward, then pulling in as you straighten and raise your arms. Stale essence flows from the arms and legs as limbs drop.
Spiritual-Emotional: Opens emotions in the chest, releases anxiety and frustration, along with stale essence and the overheated condition.
Instructions: 1. Feet shoulder-width apart, or wider. 2. Bend forward at the waist crossing your forearms and exhaling as you do. Heat and stale essence flow into the earth. 3. Straighten your body and lift your arms overhead, crossing at the wrists. 4. Let your arms fall out and down and let them swing naturally to a stop. Exhale with the sound "shoe."

Movements 34 through 44 / 103

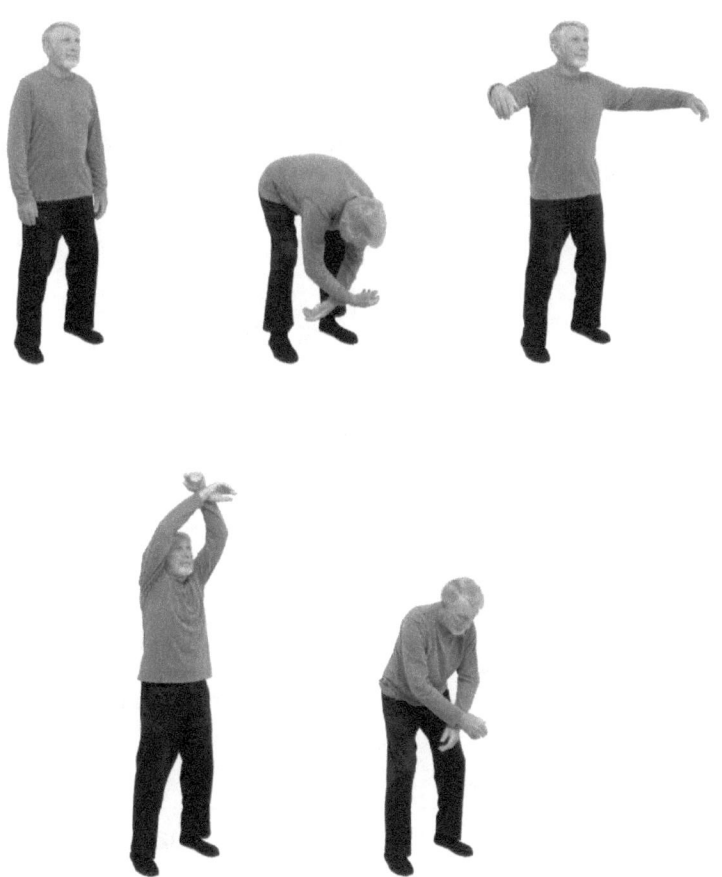

37. Sitting and Pulling the Eight Radial Cords (H)

Sowing Seeds (Y)

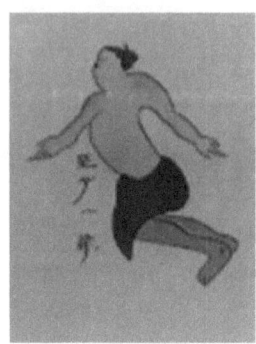

Actions: Stretching, twisting, flexibility, releasing.
Muscles: Back, shoulders, arms, legs.
Joints: Wrists, elbows, shoulders, spine, knees, ankles.
Qi Flow: Rising from the lower elixir field through the body to the fingertips and out into the cosmos; then take in *qi* through your hands to return to the lower elixir field.
Spiritual-Emotional: Centering, then expanding, connecting, and regenerating.
Instructions: 　1.　This can be done while standing or kneeling. 　2.　Start by facing South. 　3.　Feet close together, palms facing up by the lower elixir field. 　4.　Turn from the waist, while exhaling and extend your right arm as though throwing seeds from your hand. Your other hand extends gently back. 　5.　Feel stale essence being pulled from your extended hand. 　6.　Pause, to feel fresh essence being pulled into your hand. Then, gather your hands in front of the lower elixir field as you inhale.

7. Now your left arm throws seeds, as you exhale. Pause to feel the exchange of essence, then your hands return to the lower elixir field.
8. Turn 45 degrees to your right and repeat steps 4 to 7.
9. Continue turning right 45 degrees until you have faced eight directions.

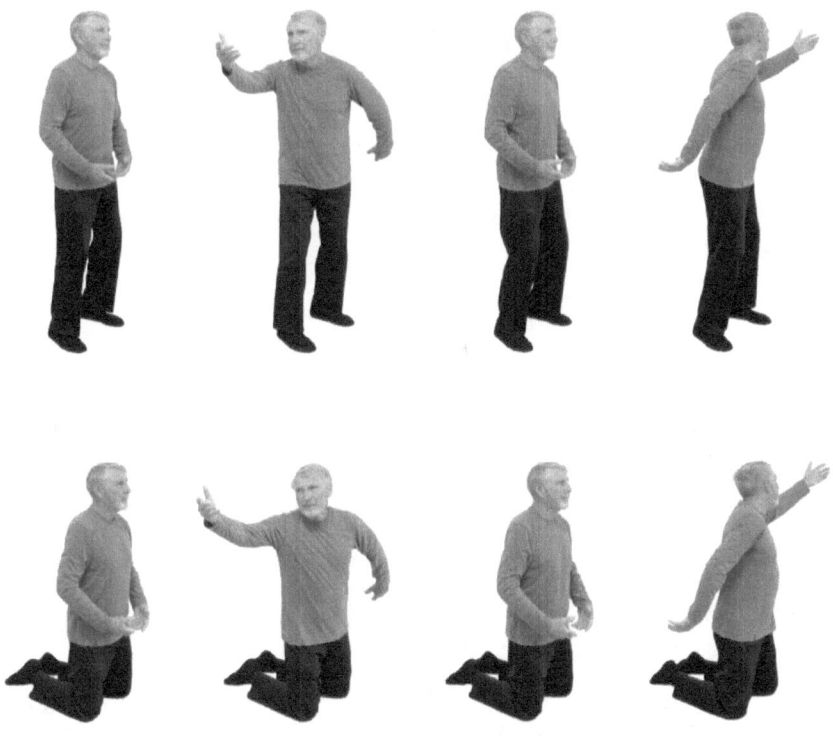

38. Praying Palms, Thrusting Elbows (A)

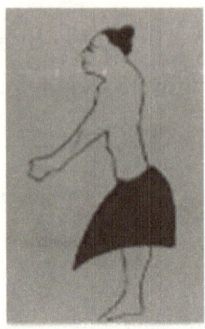

Actions: Stretching, opening and closing the torso, clearing, meditation. The picture seems to indicate abdominal compression in either inhalation or exhalation.
Muscles: Shoulders, arms, chest, diaphragm, abdominals.
Joints: Wrists, elbows, shoulders, spine.
Qi Flow: Rises from lower to middle elixir field and into chest, shoulders, arms, and hands. The flow may be up the spine or through the body. Kidneys are stimulated.
Spiritual-Emotional: Clearing or cleansing, balancing and meditation.

Instructions:
  1. Feet shoulder-width apart.
  2. Start with palms facing each other, but not quite touching, in front of your middle elixir field.
  3. Separate palms by raising both elbows to the sides up to shoulder level.
  4. As you exhale, drop both elbows and put palms back facing each other again, not quite touching.
  5. Start slowly and increase speed as desired.

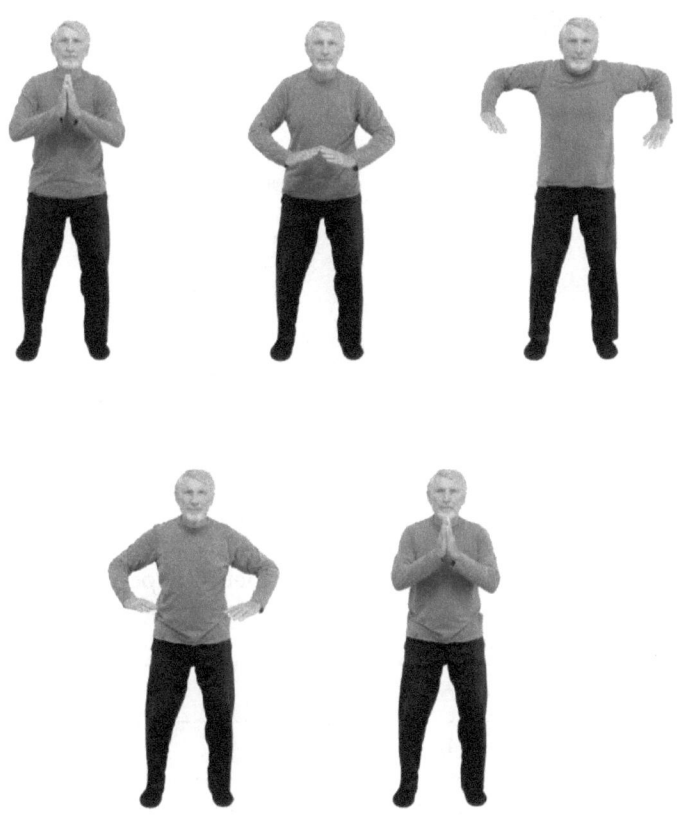

39. Pulling Ham Pain (H)

Rolling and Rocking (A)

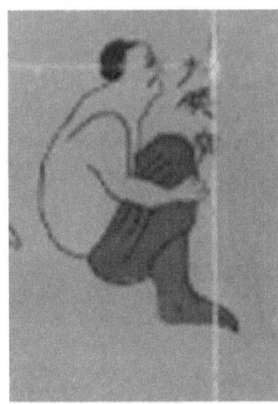

Actions: Muscle massage (including perineum), opening the sacrum.
Muscles: Gluteus, legs, back, arms.
Joints: Knees, wrists, elbows, sacroiliac.
Qi Flow: Lower elixir field to sacrum and down legs.
Spiritual-Emotional: Rocking, spiraling motion provides physical release as well as the potential to exchange pain for healing earth energy.

Instructions:
    1. Sit on the floor and grasp your shins.
    2. Turn your trunk to rock from side to side massaging your gluteus muscles.
    3. You can also massage the back muscles by leaning back.
NOTE: If you keep your knees together and place your palms on the floor beside your hips you can get a better and more controlled massage of the gluteus muscle and the sacral joint.

Movements 34 through 44 / 109

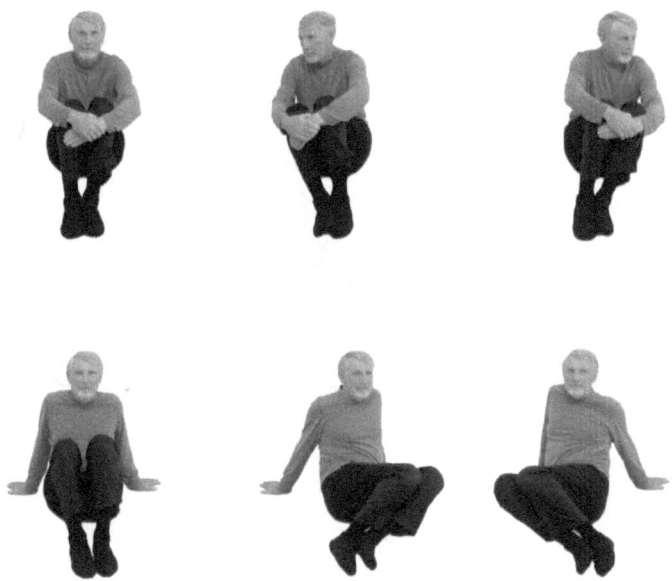

40. Gibbon Jump (K)

Gibbon Shouting (H)

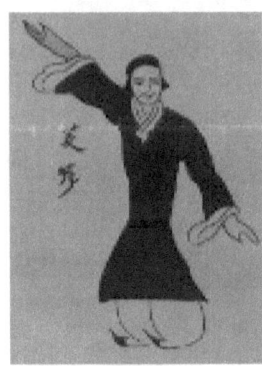

Actions: Stretching, athletic jumping (if desired).
Muscles: All.
Joints: All.
Qi Flow: Rising through the body to the hands and feet, then back to the lower elixir field.
Spiritual-Emotional: Striving, nurturing, getting rid of something unwanted, connection with the Monkey.
Instructions: 1. Feet shoulder-width apart. 2. Reach up with your right hand as though picking a piece of fruit from a tree. 3. Bring your hand to your mouth, where you pull stale essence and thrust away with your right hand (as though throwing away bitter fruit). Make a "hoo" sound as you exhale. 4. Repeat the movements with your left hand. 5. Start slowly, and if you wish you can add a small jump as though all the low-hanging fruit is gone.

Movements 34 through 44 / 111

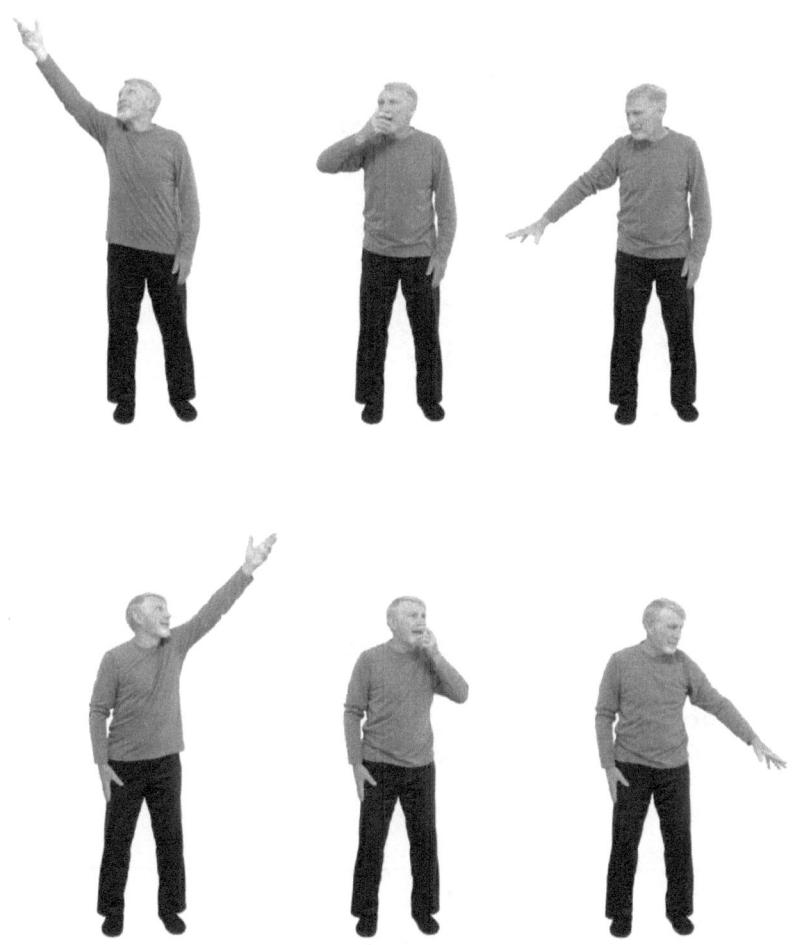

41. Bear Ramble (H)
Bear Amble (K)

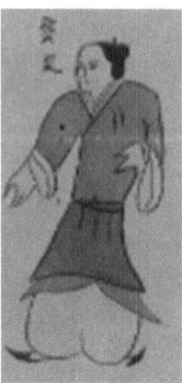

Actions: Loosening, massage of the kidneys and bladder.
Muscles: Legs, back, arms.
Joints: Hips, shoulders, spine.
Qi Flow: Moving from the lower elixir field to the sacrum, then up the back through shoulders and arms, and also flowing down the legs. It passes through the Yongquan (Bubbling Spring) points into the earth and from there rises back up the legs to the lower elixir field.
Spiritual-Emotional: Imagination, feeling of power, connection with the bear.
Instructions: 1. This movement may originally have been done with a stomping foot, but to protect knees, hips and spine, it has been modified. 2. Feet wider than shoulder-width apart, arms out from your sides as though you are a large bear. 3. Move your left arm and left leg at the same time, carefully placing your left foot down. Savor the feeling of your stale essence being exchanged for fresh essence from the earth. 4. Swing your right arm and leg around and carefully place your right foot down, savoring the feeling.

Movements 34 through 44 / 113

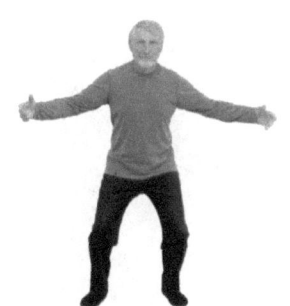

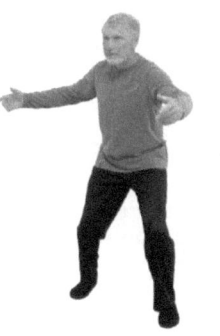

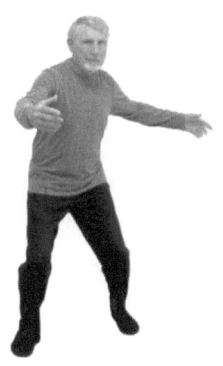

42. Turtle Move (K)

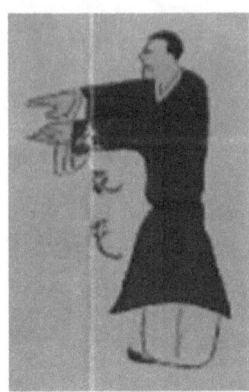

Actions: Flexibility, focusing attention and *qi*, moving meditation.
Muscles: Back, shoulders, arms, legs.
Joints: All.
Qi Flow: Places intent in Laogong points and the lower elixir field.
Spiritual-Emotional: Meditation.
Instructions: 1. Feet shoulder-width apart, or wider; your arms are just below shoulder height. 2. Imagine you have a *qi* ball between your palms with your right hand on top. 3. Keeping your hands in that position, turn at the waist to your right as far as comfortable. 4. Then, rotate your arms to place your left hand on top of the *qi* ball and turn your waist to the left. 5. Meditate, and place your heart-mind in the lower elixir field.

Movements 34 through 44 / 115

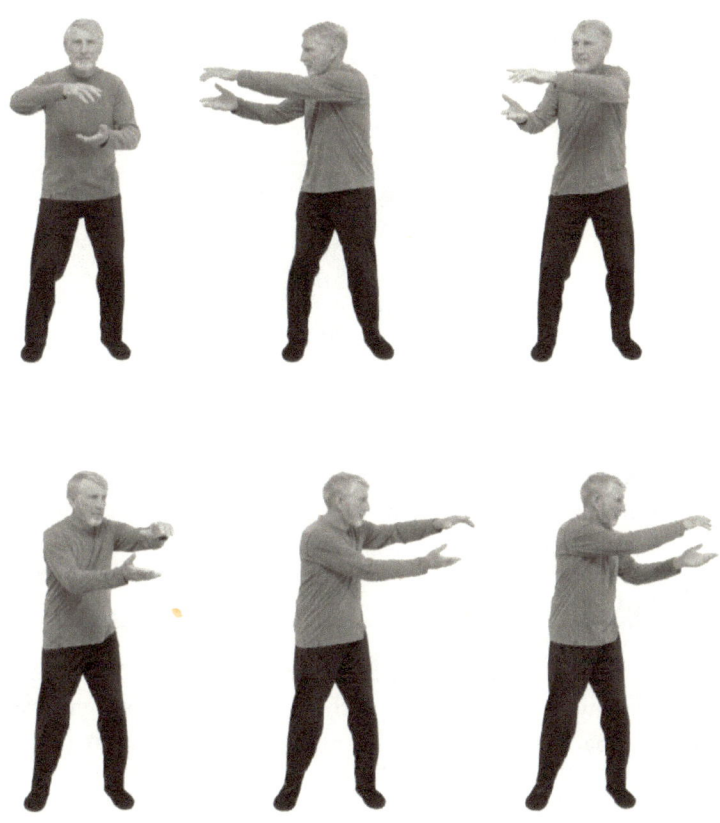

43. Turning the Wheel (A)

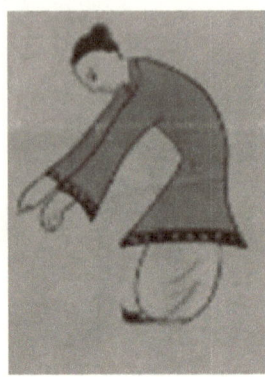

Actions: Stretching, release through large movements, coordination, uniting with *qi*. Connects with four of the six directions, north-south and up-down. (Note: #44 connects with East-West).

Muscles: All.

Joints: All.

Qi Flow: Rising from feet through the body to the top of your head and hands, then back to your feet and into the earth.

Spiritual-Emotional: Feeling of oneness; full opening of body and connection of personal *qi* with energy all around.

Instructions:
1. Feet shoulder-width apart, or wider, palms above your shoulders, facing forward. Do slowly, relishing each movement.
2. Reach upward and when at full extension bring your arms outward and downward toward the earth.
3. Bring your hands straight up your sides.
4. Repeat, as you gather *qi* from four directions.
5. Perform this movement in reverse to expel stale essence through your hands and feet as you squat.

6. Bring your hands and arms forward as in Yang-style "lifting water" as you straighten your legs and your arms, then bring your hands down the sides of your body to the earth.

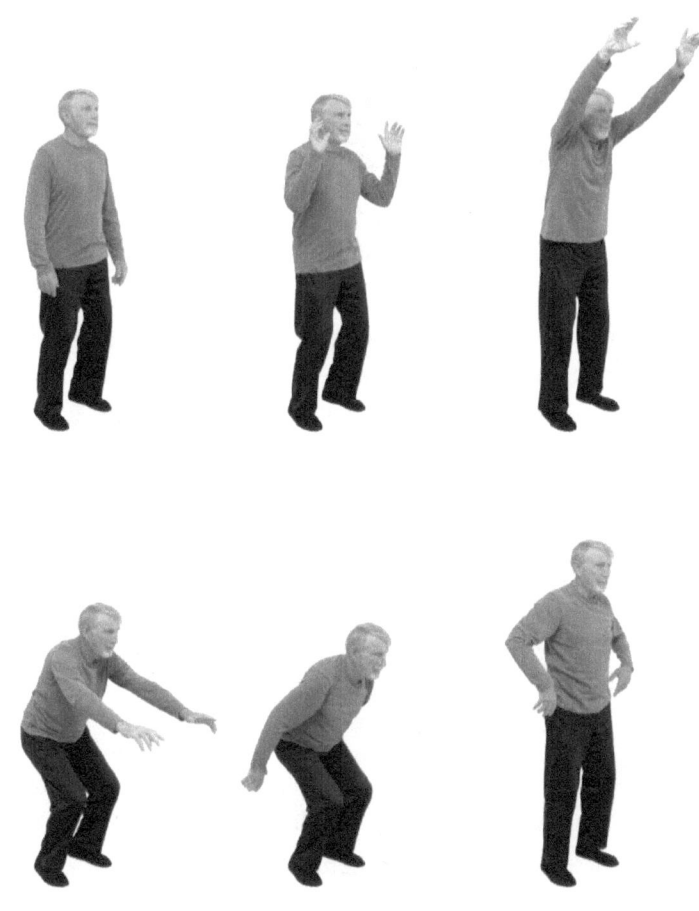

44. Merlin (H)

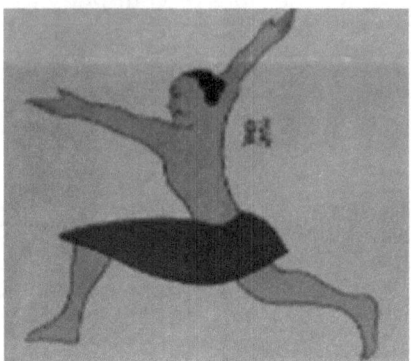

Actions: Stretching, release, balance, imagery. Connects with East and West, completing the last two of the six directions. This could have been considered a demonstration of overall flexibility, balance, and health.
Muscles: All.
Joints: All.
Qi Flow: Balanced.
Spiritual-Emotional: Release, emergence, a Merlin is a type of falcon, so you can imagine you are a soaring bird.
Instructions: 　1. Feet wider than shoulder-width apart. The reconstructed picture resembles a yoga warrior II pose, but this movement has more of a flying dynamic, hence the name Merlin. 　2. Spread your arms like wings, step 45 degrees to the left with your left leg. 　3. Turn your torso to the left, bend and move your left hand toward your left foot, as in a Yang style taijiquan low single whip. 　4. Straighten your right leg and bend your left knee, while extending the left arm with fingers at eye-level. Then bring your right arm around to join the left.

5. Turn your body to the right, bringing your right hand down toward your right foot. Raise your right arm, with fingers at eye-level, then move your left hand to join the right. Now you are facing to the right with both arms extended and fingers at eye-level.

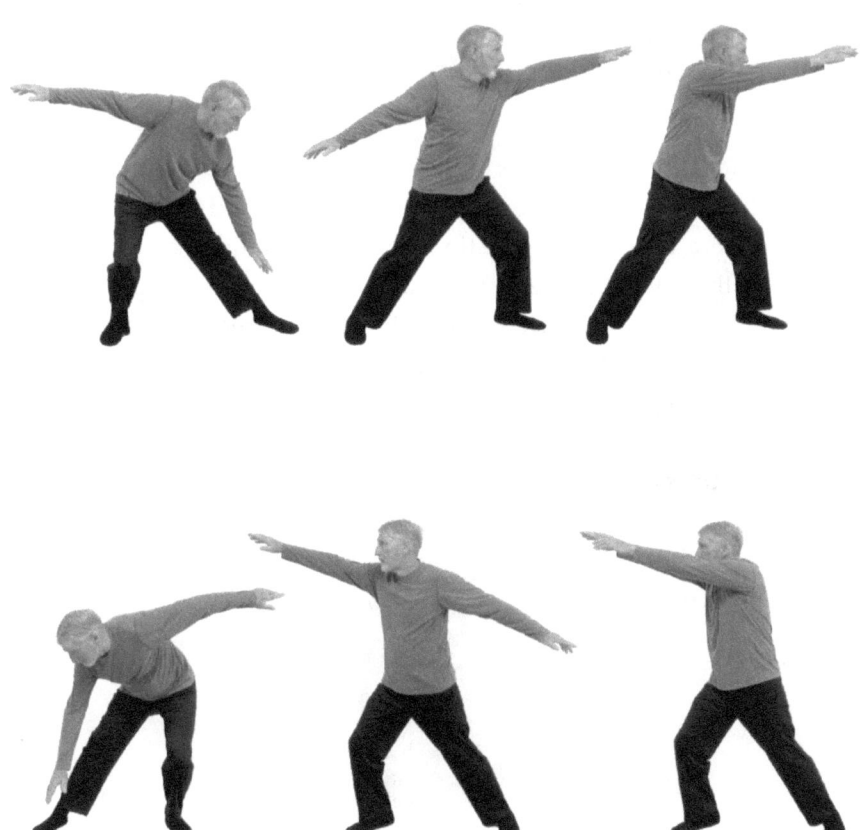

Chapter Eight

Interpretations and Combinations

Chang Tsao, a well-known painter of the Tang period said: "Outwardly I follow the creativity of nature; inwardly I gain from the source of my heart."

To follow the law of nature is to be free from human limitations and confining rules. To obtain something from the source of one's heart is the process of self-realization. (Chang 2011, 247)

The *Daoyintu* provided a pictorial list of treatment options from which shaman-physicians could choose one or more that would apply. It is likely that there were different applications, or interpretations of the images, even when they were in their original, complete forms. Applying the concept of the uncarved block, we were inspired to create different meanings for images: #24, #41, #38, and #42. Additionally, we combined multiple *daoyin* movements to create three purposeful forms.

The Pace of Yu

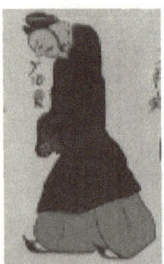

Fig. 8: *Daoyintu* #24

As noted in Chapter Six above, *Daoyintu* #24 has a legible Chinese name or purpose of "Pulling an Upper Side Accumulation," which, according to Donald Harper, is a way to relieve a "vapor" (*qi*) blockage. Every aspect of this figure portrays a walking meditation or prayer. The authors think this drawing could depict the Pace of Yu, a stylized form of stepping that was used by shaman-physicians in many ancient rituals.

The Pace of Yu is named in reference to the Great Yu, the mythical Chinese hero who controlled the flood waters (Despeux 2004, 74). Donald Harper writes that the Pace of Yu appears eight times in magical recipes unearthed at Mawangdui. He states: "The earliest occurrence of the term was in the *Shizi* (pre-Han), in a description of the physical deformities suffered by Yu (the hero of the Chinese flood myth and legendary founder of the Xia ruling house)" (2009, 167-8). This was a ritual act usually performed at the beginning of a magical activity, often with an incantation. At some point, the Pace of Yu became part of Daoist practice.

Note that right foot of the practitioner in #24 is forward. This is significant because it marks the starting position of the Pace of Yu. Its performance, as Donald Harper describes it, is as follows:

> Beginning with the right foot in front and the left foot behind, the performer steps ahead with the left foot and then again with the right foot, finally bringing the left foot even with the right foot—which concludes the first pace. The second pace continues by stepping ahead with the right foot, followed by the left foot, finally bringing the right foot even with the left foot. The third pace repeats the first pace. (Harper 2009, 169)

The authors have modified the original footwork instructions by adding breathing advice. Here is our version:

Pace of Yu
1. Start with your right foot forward. Breathe in as you lift your left heel.
2. Step ahead with your left foot, breathing out as your left heel touches the earth.
3. Then step ahead with your right foot, breathing in as you lift your right heel and out, as your right heel touches the earth.

> 4. Bring (shuffle) your left foot even with your right foot. (This is the first Pace.)
> 5. Step ahead with your right foot and then ahead with your left foot.
> 6. Bring (shuffle) your right foot even with your left foot. (This is the second Pace.)
> 7. Repeat 2-4 for the third Pace and 4-6 for the fourth Pace, etc.

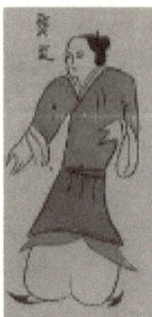

Fig. 9: *Daoyintu* #41

Moving on, #41, Bear Ramble, may also have been performed with footwork similar to the Pace of Yu, as it is said Yu dressed like a bear. "But Yu also dressed up as a bear and, in some measure, incarnated the Bear Spirit" (Eliade 2004, 458).

If you apply the Pace of Yu to Bear Ramble, you maintain a wide stance and move the whole side of your body with each step. Take the time to feel exchange of stale essence for fresh essence through each foot.

Standing Meditation

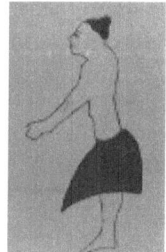

Fig. 10: *Daoyintu* #38

Daoyintu #38 is one of the incomplete drawings. Only the top half of the image is visible in the original silk painting, and so it is unclear whether the legs should straight or bent. There is no writing associated with the image, so it is nameless. The figure's arms are bare, and he possibly has no shirt, which could indicate that he is a martial figure.

The authors think that #38 depicts a form of standing meditation, similar to what is today called Standing Posture (*zhanzhuang*), also rendered Standing Pole or Standing Like a Tree. It is an outwardly simple posture in which you stand still while the *qi* works within. Well-known as a martial art exercise, the idea of standing meditation goes back at least as far as the medical classic *Huangdi neijing* and the ancient Daoist *Daodejing*.

> In the "Plain Questions" section of the *Inner Classic of the Yellow Emperor* (ca. 3rd c. BCE), we read that the ancients would "support heaven and earth, taking hold of yin and yang, breathing the air of vitality *(jingqi)*, standing alone guarding their spirit *(shen)*, the muscles as one." This passage, though clearly open to interpretation, strongly suggests the practice of a static standing exercise to nurture tranquility and health. (Wang and Moffett 1994, 29)

Chapter 16 in the *Daodejing* translation by Hua-Ching Ni similarly suggests a form of standing meditation:

Attain utmost unoccupiedness.
Maintain the utmost stillness,
And do not interfere with all the things
That rush together in activity and grow luxuriantly,
Then you can see how living things flourish
And renew themselves.
Yet, they must all return to the root again,
Each to its simple source.
Knowing to return to the root is to be refreshed.
This is called subtle revitalization.
To restore one's vitality is to constantly renew oneself. (2003, 25)

If we were to draw the front view of a Standing Posture, it might look very similar to #41. However, the latter is named Bear Ramble, so it clearly is not a static posture. #38 itself gives the impression of being static, as do the other still meditational figures in #3 and 19.

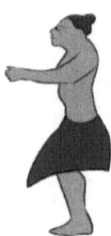

Fig. 11: Modified *Daoyintu* #38

Standing Posture`
1. Relax into a Horse Stance. A horse stance is wider than a Wuji stance, with your legs farther apart and knees bent, as though you were riding a horse.
2. Let your muscles relax and follow your breath, while allowing your *qi* to move.
3. Lift your arms.
4. Soften your breathing, clear your mind, and nurture yourself.

If you have practiced Standing Posture, you know this already and can read more about it elsewhere (e.g., see Lam 1991; Wang and Moffett 1994), since an in-depth discussion is beyond the scope of this book.

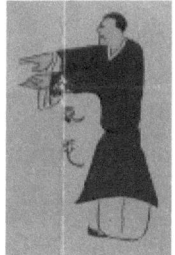

Fig. 12: *Daoyintu* #42

The image of *Daoyintu* #42 is quite clear in the original manuscript. Livia Kohn writes that it is called Turtle Move, however, there is no consensus among scholars that this is the name of the image. Despite that lack of academic agreement, the idea of a turtle move is appealing. Turtle or tortoise shells, carved with symbols, were used thousands of years ago in China, both for divination and to express wishes.

> The kings of the late Shang (ca/ 1200-1050 BCE.) attempted to communicate with the spiritual forces that rule their world by reading the stress cracks in cattle bones and turtle plastrons. They and their diviners produced these cracks by applying a heated brand or poker to the consecrated bones or shells, intoning as they did so a charge that conveyed their intentions, wishes, or need to know. (Ebrey 1995, 3)

Tortoise Insight
1. Assume the posture of *Daoyintu* #42.
2. The instructions for this movement in Chapter 6 are to cultivate a ball of *qi* between your hands.
3. After you have done this for some time, imagine a tortoise shell, carved with mystical symbols, between your hands.

> 4. As you move the shell from side to side, it may put you in touch with things that are meaningful to you, and that may give you insights.

Combinations

Here are several forms used by the authors. Note that the order of performing the movements they depict is from left to right.

1. Simply Guiding and Pulling Stale Essence

Daoyintu #9 and 14 complement each other. Movement #9 guides and pulls stale essence out, as your arms thrust outward or downward. #14 pulls in and guides fresh essence as your arms reach out and your palms are pulled toward the lower elixir field.

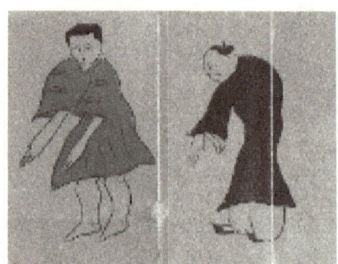

Fig. 13: *Daoyintu* #9 and 14

2. Full Release

Following the directions in previous chapters, and doing them in this sequence, releases stale essence from the body.

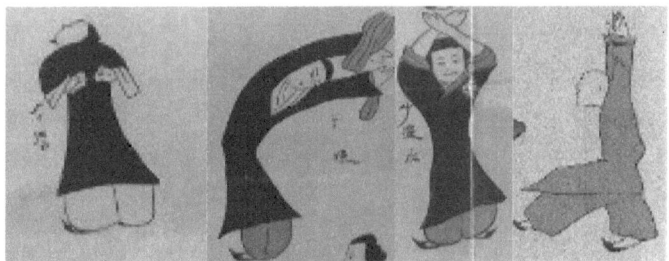

Fig. 14: *Daoyintu* #2, 8, 36, 12

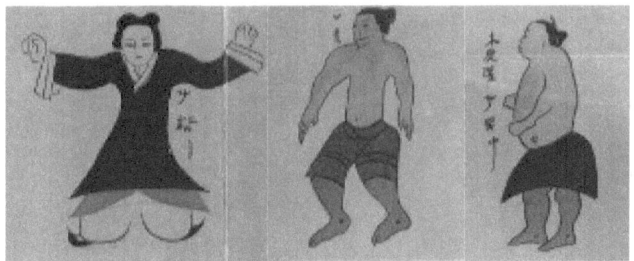

Fig. 15: *Daoyintu* #20, 15, 35

Full Release
1. #2 Release stale essence with your exhalation.
2. #8 Praying Mantis: Guide and pull stale essence, releasing through the finger wells.
3. #36 Pulling the Warm Ailment and expelling into the earth.
4. #12 Giant Step: Guide and pull stale essence to your arms and expel through your fingers as you step forward.
5. #20 Pulling Deafness (Bear Drops). Release stale essence and fear into the earth.
6. #15 Pulling Inguinal Swelling: Guide and pull stale essence, which is released through your fingers and feet as your body drops.
7. #35 Monkey Bawling: Release heat and emotions through your breath and bouncing.

128 / Chapter Eight

3. Shamanic Form

Shaman-healers had a spiritual relationship with animals that is not easy to appreciate today. Yet by becoming as the uncarved block, clearing and opening your mind, and suspending disbelief, one can hope to experience a spiritual relationship.

> It has been demonstrated that ancient China felt a relationship, charged with a highly complex cosmological and initiatory symbolism, between the shamanic dance and an animal. (Eliade 2004, 458-59)

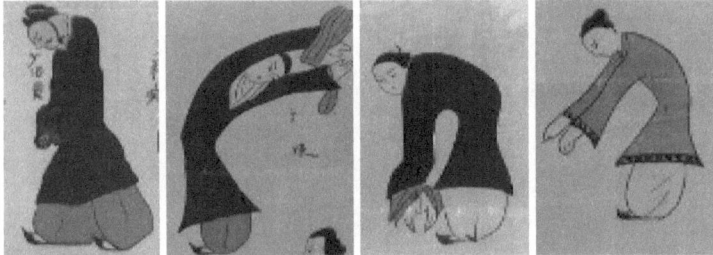

Fig. 16: *Daoyintu* #24, 8, 1, 43

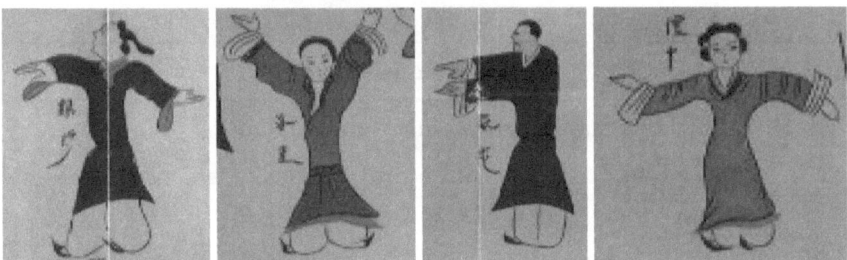

Fig. 17: *Daoyintu* #25, 27, 42, 18

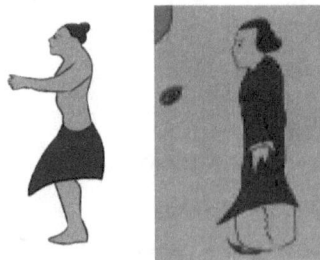

Fig. 18: *Daoyintu* #38, 19

Shamanic Form

1. #24, Pace of Yu: Walk the seven-star pattern of the Big Dipper, while cherishing yourself, and ending by facing north. State your wishes for improving your health. Now turn south and engrave your wishes on a tortoise shell.
2. #8, Praying Mantis: Pulling and guiding to release and clear with this movement.
3. #1, Opening to heaven and earth: Connecting with both.
4. #43, Turning the Wheel: Guide and pull *qi* from the universe.
5. #25, Crane Call: Open yourself to the spirit of the crane.
6. #27, Dragon Ascending: Invite the spirit of the dragon to give you power.
7. #42, Turtle Move: In your hands is a symbolic, engraved tortoise shell. Combine your intent to be healthy, and your cherished self, with your *qi*, which you place inside the shell. Let it become a healing talisman that you use for self-massage to apply as your intuition guides you.
8. #18, Inside the Abdomen: Pull (roll) a ball of *qi* externally from hand to hand, while your *qi* moves inside you
9. #38, Standing Meditation: Stand or sit in tree hugging position to allow the *qi* to seek its own balance.
10. #19, Centered Breathing: Meditate while standing or seated.

Chapter Nine
Self and Self-Care

We consider the exercises outlined in the *Daoyintu* as a complementary health practice, mostly done for well-being. However, there also may be times when we do them to alleviate disease, defined as follows:

> The source of disease is any challenge of the body with which it is unable to cope, whether it is a harmful substance or a bad feeling. Disease is a manifestation of an unstable process, a pattern of disharmonious relationships. When defenses are weakened and resources exhausted a multiplicity of factors conspire to permit illness. (Beinfeld and Korngold 1991, 36)

As you embark on complementary health practices, continue to follow the treatments that your medical professionals have advised. Do not estrange yourself from outside support. Still accept the advice of family, associates, and medical teams as well as share your complementary health activities with them. Keep firmly in mind that you are considering methods of self-care to augment any treatments you already receive.

Proposed Self-Care Approach

Practitioners of traditional Chinese medicine often make a contract with a patient because a specific commitment increases the likelihood of successful treatment. Caroline Myss defines such a contract as "two parties agreeing to participate in some task or to hold themselves accountable for the same commitments, for a mutually beneficial reason" (2003, 48).

In the acupuncture clinic, the consultation sheet is the written contract and the patient and the practitioner are two equal parties seeking a resolution to a primary concern about well-being via a conferred treatment plan. Annie Mitchell and Maggie Mc Cormack write:

Practical action provides the means by which the practitioner can empower the patient, to help him towards understanding what he can do to cope with his illness. Attention to the patient's own possibilities for action and self-care provide a balance in treatment away from dependency, or professional powerful control, towards enhancing the patient's own sense of personal power and self-efficacy. (This is) the heart of therapeutic encounter. (1998, 40)

By initiating a dialogue with yourself, you can create a self-care plan to augment your other treatments with activities from the *Daoyintu*.

Introspection and Personal Candor

Self-diagnosis doesn't come easily. Putting yourself in a receptive state of mind for introspection, personal candor, and creativity is crucial to getting the most of this process.

We offer a simple ritual to help put you in this receptive state, and perhaps experience the inspiration of ancient Chinese shaman-physi-cians who practiced ritual as an indispensable part of their medical theory and practice.

When you are ready to begin the work on your very own personal self-care contract, get ready by following these instructions.

Preparation
1. Sit down.
2. Lower your eyes.
3. Listen to your heart beat.
4. Breathe in the mood of ambience that surrounds you.
5. Smile into your lower, middle, and upper elixir fields to align the Three Treasures, essence, *qi*, and spirit.
6. Meditate on why you are here.

Once you have put yourself in a calm yet ready state, you are well on your way to an assessment of your state of health and an openness to your body's wisdom. Be open-minded, non-judgmental. You may be conscious of other presences: prepare to be receptive.

Here is an example of a questionnaire that forms the basis of a self-care contract. You can use it to help you find what you want and need, then create a plan of action to augment treatments you already receive.

My Self-Care Contract

The purpose of this form is to help you determine if and how you may supplement your medical treatments with *daoyin*.

Section 1: Reflect

Start by mentally scanning yourself from head to toe, noting your external and internal state. Have a dialogue with yourself and write down your responses on a piece of paper or in a special notebook.

1. What is my present state of health?
2. Do I have a diagnosed condition that concerns me?
3. Are there other conditions that I feel have not been addressed?
4. What changes do I want to achieve?

Section 2: Assess Emotions

Answer the following questions:

1. What emotions weaken me?
2. What emotions give me confidence and strength?
3. Am I filling myself with positive emotions?
4. Am I turning my attention within?

Section 3: Intuition

You can explore your intuition by reflecting on these issues:

1. Does an internal whisper speak to me about improving my condition?
2. Is there a guide or angel, or inner doctor to ask as well?

Write down any feedback you receive or impressions you have.

Section 4: Use *Daoyintu* Figures

Visualize the *Daoyintu* figures as uncarved blocks, then reflect on the following questions:

1. Which figures appeal or speak or call to me?
2. Do I want to become one or more of the figures?
3. How do I envision the guiding and pulling of energy?

Section 5: Affirm Attention

Use your answers to these many questions as a guideline, adding items as you desire. When you feel your session is over, you will hopefully have insight, a way ahead, and a vision of your future self who is balanced and healthy. Your insights may be direct and prescriptive, or symbolic, or you may not perceive any recognizable message at the time. Sometimes, the insight can manifest itself suddenly, hours, or even days later.

Select the *Daoyintu* movements or forms that you think best apply to your situation. Here are some methods to try for inspiration.

---

1. As you were reading this book and learning how to perform the *Daoyintu* movements, you may have consciously selected some that you feel are beneficial. By all means do them now, whether single movements or one of the forms.
2. There were probably some movements you simply enjoyed doing and perhaps some that you didn't like. Do at least three of

your favorite movements. Then do three of your least favorite ones.

3. Place a copy of the *Daoyintu* figures on a table, close your eyes and allow your subconscious mind to work. Move your finger over the drawing until you are inclined to stop. Do the movement or movements as indicated by your spontaneous choice(s).

4. Prepare yourself to channel not just the behavior of an animal or animals, but their spirit as well. Ready yourself, if you wish, to take your own shamanic journey.

5. Mentally trace images of any of the *Daoyintu* figures that come to mind on the "uncarved block." Superimpose yourself on the image. Allow your body to relax, let your mind follow your breath, and immerse yourself in a sacred space of harmony and light.

Best establish a schedule to undertake the activities and perform the movements that apply to your situation. Daily is a good place to start.

Finally, a strong statement of personal commitment can be useful as a motivator. If you write or articulate a heart-felt intention, you will be that much more likely to follow through on your chosen course of action. Ask yourself: Can I visualize or do I have a safe place which gives me peace and solace in times of distress or discomfort? How can I prepare myself for that sacred space?

Chapter Ten

Initiating Engagement

In this chapter, we move away from interpretation of history, health exercise, and self-analysis into less travelled regions. Here we share methods to cleanse ourselves and our practice area, and then open ourselves to the possibility of mystical, even ecstatic experiences in our energy work.

How many times during periods of frustration have we raised our hands above our head and, with a deep sigh, thrown our arms out in a gesture of disgust to cast out a troubling issue. This deep sigh is a type of relieving exhale. We do the same when we yawn to release stale *qi* from the liver. Then, we naturally take in a "breath of fresh air." Both are similar natural processes and require little if any effort to invigorate ourselves with revitalizing *qi*.

Cleansing Breath

There are a number of different methods of cleansing, one of which is through the breath. Tsung-Hwa Jou describes it as "inhaling through the nose and exhaling through the mouth" (1981, 124). Here is an example of cleansing breath based upon an actual experience that was personally witnessed in Tainan, Taiwan, early one morning in 1972.

There was the staccato sound of a motorcycle sputtering as it moved on the sandy road. A slightly opened garden gate showed the figure of a burly man jolting his motor cycle to a sudden stop in the early dawn light. He slid from the seat of his bike and spat a curse at the neighbor's house across the way. He clumsily began to unstrap a huge boulder which sank the rear tire of the motorcycle deep into the road. He hugged the boulder and struggled to hoist it to his chest. He staggered and grunted as he carried it toward his neighbor's gate. He heaved. With a loud shout, he crashed the boulder into the gate next door. Relieved of his burden, the man slapped his hands together in a moment of victorious release. He smiled and mounted his bike with a wide straddle. He drove away straight backed and proud.

The principal point to be gained from this story is that some of the concepts of ancient cleansing rituals have persisted through the ages. They have become inherently a part of the thoughts and actions of those who either consciously or unconsciously practice them. We may surmise that the protagonist in the story cleansed himself of anger and anxiety by releasing them to the exterior, with his shouting breath, rather than harboring them internally.

Ritual

We have noted that ritual can touch hidden archetypal forces and may induce dynamic therapeutic change within us.

We regularly augment our *daoyin* activities by using personal, sometimes Daoist-inspired ritual. This has a long history. As Livia Kohn points out: "As healing exercises became a part of Daoist practices, they were formalized in the priestly hierarchy of Tang Daoism, introduced with ritual formalities and transmitted in ordination-type ceremonies" (2008, 158).

We consider ritual to be an essential adjunct to the preparation for, and practice of, energy work. Our rituals center upon preparing ourselves and creating sacred healing space to practice *daoyin*. We have used all the methods presented here, but they are meant as inspiring examples or models, not strict dogmas to be followed without question. You may find other rituals that serve you better to add to the preparatory arrangements described below.

Historically, facing south is the favored position of practice: it means being in line with the emperor facing yang or south with his back toward cold yin in the north (Maciocia 1989, 5). The direction we face during practice may involve sampling expert advice (see examples in App. 3), but ultimately the choice of direction to face is up to you and your environment. One of the authors had a student who did her healing meditation in a small walk-in closet, with limited choice of direction to face, because it was the only private space available. The authors recommend facing south when possible.

Another powerful ritual is found in ringing bells, which Daoists used for celebrations as well as to drive out evil from their temples. In Tainan (Taiwan), some Daoist priests walk in a crooked path while ringing bells in order to evade and befuddle the demons, who are confined to walking a straight line. A bell or gong, then, can help clear your room.

Candles similarly can be used to represent yin and yang, for example: a black candle matches yin, the moon, and the earth, while a white one relates to yang, the sun, and the heavens. Cinnabar-red candles symbolize oneness with Dao. The flame and glow of any candle can enhance ambiance.

Beyond that, you may also wish to prepare an herbal infusion of your choice to take into your healing space. Herbs such as thyme and sage have healing qualities and help create an environment of healing whether consumed, burned at an altar, or ceremoniously used to massage and cleanse the body, to awaken, or soothe senses. "Sage is extremely beneficial to the system as a whole" (Soo 1986, 54). The "[*Huangdi*] *Neijing* itself mentions only roots, stalks, and the topmost branches of thyme" (Veith 1949, 55).

Divine Connections

There are many Daoist deities, some that have existed since the beginning of time, called gods of precreation or "former heaven" (*xiantian*) and those who came later, called deities after creation or "later heaven" (*houtian*) (Wong 1997, 146-59). Some reside in stars or constellations, such as the Big Dipper, and some are associated with each of the directions.

Khigh Alx Dhiegh presents a list of mythical starry emperors in relation to the five phases, the seasons, and the directions.

Taihao	Wood	Spring	East
Yandi	Fire	Summer	South
Huangdi	Earth	Late Summer	Center
Shaohao	Metal	Autumn	West
Chuanxu	Water	Winter	North (Dhiegh 1973. 47)

You may find one deity, or several, who appeal to you.

Shamanic spiritual and healing practices are implied in the *Daoyintu* and explicit in other documents that accompanied it in the Mawangdui tomb. Some shamanic practices may be appealing as you seek connection to a healing presence. The *Daoyintu* contains movements associated with animals such as the mantis, monkey, crane, dragon tiger, bear, turtle, and merlin. Dressing or behaving like an animal was a common element in the shamanistic practices of many countries' cultures, including ancient China.

> The important thing is what they (shamans) felt when they masqueraded as animals. We have reason to believe that this magical transformation resulted in a 'going out of the self' that very often found expression in an ecstatic experience. (Eliade 2004, 459)

Doing the movements of an animal, can lift one's spirit, and may even contribute to an ecstatic out-of-body experience.

By recognizing these divine connections prior to doing *daoyin*, a practitioner may become attuned with the ancient Daoist milieu and perhaps resonate with beneficial deities or animals.

Proper Preparation

We suggest the following three rituals just prior to entering your sacred space so that there is a distinct break between the matters of your daily life and your special practice.

Abstain

Fast for an hour, or more, before embarking on a serious *daoyin* session. You should neither be distracted by being too hungry, nor too full. Be aware that your spirituality can be enhanced by a degree of abstention.

Cleanse

This includes body and emotional/spiritual cleansing. Wash your face and hands with warm soap and water. If water is not available, you may wish to physically rub your torso and limbs with a dry wash. Rinse your mouth with warm water or tea to clear any sour, bitter, sweet, or pungent taste.

Here is a variation of *Daoyintu* 12, that we call Boulder Breathing, for the purpose of cleansing. You may, of course, augment or replace this with emotional and spiritual cleansing actions of your choice.

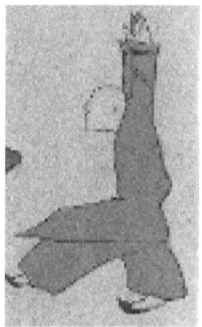

Figure 19: *Daoyintu* 12

Boulder Breathing
1. Face an open space.
2. Squat down to the floor with knees bent in a lifting position that is comfortable for you.
3. Wrap your arms around an imaginary large boulder that contains emotions you want to expel.
4. Inhale deeply as you lift the imaginary boulder over your head.
5. Throw the boulder away from you, while you step and exhale with a forceful shout.
6. Repeat until lifting and throwing the boulder is no longer a burden and your negative emotions are dispelled.

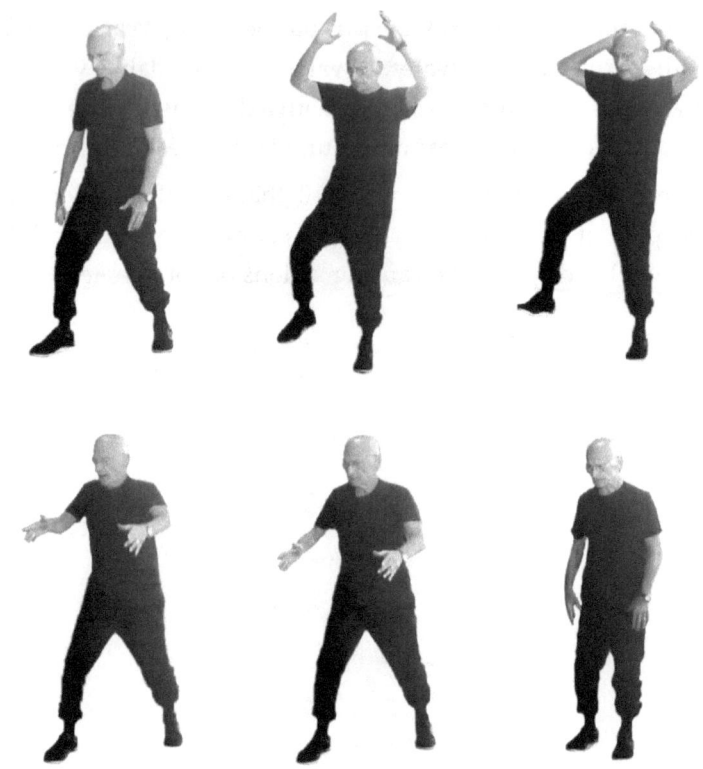

Affirm

Review your Self-Care Contract.

Repeat the names of your infirmities.

Resolve to face their root cause.

Invoke the enlightening power of virtue (*de*).

Smile.

Inhale deeply.

Softly exhale the fading past. Put the cares of the world behind you.

You are now ready to enter your sacred space.

Chapter Eleven

Your *Daoyintu* Experience

Having prepared a sanctum and yourself, you are on the threshold of a very personal experience with the *Daoyintu*—one in which your intuition and imagination come into play. Your intentions may vary, ranging from simply stretching to enhancing your state of wellness.

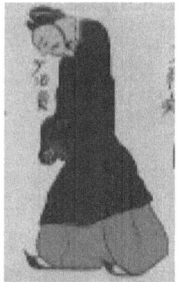

Figure 20: *Daoyintu 24*

Step into your sacred space with reverence.

Inhale slowly as your raise each heel.

Softly exhale as you take each step until you feel you are in the right place for you.

Lower your eyes.

Listen to your heart beat.

Breathe in the mood of ambience that surrounds you.

Hesitate for a moment.

Why are you here?

142 / Chapter Eleven

Incantation

Say your name.

Say your commitment.

Say *Wo shi daoyin* ("I am *daoyin*").

I have unlocked the Door.

I have entered the Space.

I have cleared the Room.

I have rung the Bell.

I have lit the Candles.

I have burnt the Incense.

I touch the Channels.

I unlock the Senses.

I feel my Pulse.

I ravish the Mood.

Let the Uncarved Block appear before me.

Let the images fly free.

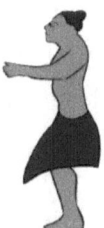

Figure 21: Modified *Daoyintu* 38

Inspirational *Daoyintu*
1. Stand in the position of #38. Make an intentional connection of your body with heaven and earth, by aligning your perineum, your spine, and the top of your head on one vertical axis.
2. Believe in your own abilities, insights, and intuition.
3. It is time to let your creative spirit guide your body in the movements of the *Daoyintu*. This is the culmination of what you have learned and practiced.
4. Mentally, or with your hands, trace images of any of the *Daoyintu* figures that come to mind on the "uncarved block." Superimpose yourself on the image you have traced. Allow your body to relax, let your mind follow your breath, and simply wait for your body and spirit to enact your inspiration.
5. Feel the *qi* within you that seeks to come out and *qi* outside you that wants to enter; it seeks to achieve an equilibrium through your breathing, through many points in your body, and finally, your entire skin. Be aware of this as you breathe and exchange *qi* with the universe.

This could take a while.

Be patient.

When the movements come, enjoy doing them. It is not uncommon to feel that the movements are doing you. There may be an urge to repeat a movement, or movements, many times and that is fine, because repetition builds energy. Your experiences may vary greatly and be quite personal.

When you feel you are finished with your *Daoyintu* experience, be sure to spend some time in seated meditation to allow your energy, body, and emotions to rebalance themselves.

You can return to your sacred space and *Daoyintu* practice any time you want.

Appendices

Appendix 1: The *Daoyintu* Movements through History

Dating from roughly the same time period as the *Daoyintu* is a medical manuscript, called *Yinshu* (Pulling Book [Lo 2014]; Stretch Book [Kohn 2008], which was excavated in 1983 from a tomb at Zhangjiashan. (Harper 2009, 31-33). The 113 bamboo strips of the *Yinshu* contain written descriptions of exercise routines for general purposes and also for specific ailments. In her translation of the *Yinshu*, Vivienne Lo writes that in five cases, similar names in *Yinshu* and the *Daoyintu* are not representative of the same exercise or treatment activity. These are bamboo strips, #28, 31, 45, 72, and 90 (2014, 42, 48, 62, 90, 104).

Some possible correlations are *Yinshu* #22 and *Daoyintu* #9; *Yinshu* #23 and *Daoyintu* #34; *Yinshu* #27 and *Daoyintu* #32; and *Yinshu* #67 and *Daoyintu* #30.

A famous set of exercises, called The Five Animals' Play (or Frolic), is attributed to Hua Tuo, a physician who lived toward the end of the Han dynasty (25-220 CE). A rare copy of the exercises inscribed on a piece of brocade has been handed down since the 10th century as an heirloom in Shen Shou's family in Zhejiang province. It bears the words, "A Genuine Heritage from Hua Tuo" (Wu and Mao 1992, 68-77).

A number of the figures portrayed there are quite reminiscent of the *Daoyintu*. Specifically, page 75 shows a figure similar to *Daoyintu* #41, page 76 shows one close to *Daoyintu* #6, and page 77 has something quite like *Daoyintu* #28.

Sun Simiao was a physician in the Tang Dynasty. who lived from 581 to 682 CE. He was the author of 30-volumes called *Qianjin yaofang* (Essential Prescriptions Worth a Thousand Pieces of Gold). An excerpt from these volumes is given in *An Illustrated Handbook of Chinese Qigong Forms* (Li 2010, 34-35). It has three descriptions that closely parallel the *Daoyintu* movements #2, 4, and 5.

Another famous set of health exercises is known as the Eight Pieces of Brocade. A representation, taken from the *Daoshu* (Pivot of Dao), compiled during the Southern Song Dynasty (1127-1279), shows *Daoyintu* movements #4, 22, 3, and 15. (Wu and Mao 1992, 110-17).

A book of martial health exercises depicts another set of Brocade movements similar to *Daoyintu* #4 and 10 (Tung 1981, 9). A different set in the same book shows movements similar to *Daoyintu* #20 and 43 (1981, 128).

During the Ming dynasty, Luo Hongxian edited a book of exercises called "Forty-Nine Prescriptions Left by the Immortals." *Daoyintu* #28 appears on page 131 and #9 is found on page 135 (Li and Zhu 2010, 130-35).

In addition, *Daoyintu* #39 appears in *The Complete System of Self-Healing* by Dr. Stephen T. Chang (1986, 153).

All this means that nearly a third of the *Daoyintu* movements have persisted through the centuries, more specifically #2, 3, 4, 5, 6, 9, 10, 15, 20, 22, 28, 32, 39, 41, and 43.

Appendix 2: Five Phases Correspondence Chart[1]

	Water	Wood	Fire	Earth	Metal
Season	Winter	Spring	Summer	Late Sum	Autumn
Climate	Cold	Wind	Heat	Dampness	Dryness
Yang Organ	Bladder	Gall-bladder	Small Intestine	Stomach	Large Intestine
Yin Organ	Kidney	Liver	Heart	Spleen	Lung
Sense	Ears	Eyes	Tongue	Mouth	Nose

---

[1] This chart is a composite, taken from various sources, including Kit 2002, 45; Chia and Chia 2007, 68; and Lau 1990, 26.

Body Tissue	Bone	Sinews	Blood Vessel	Muscles Flesh	Skin/Hair
Negative Emotion	Fear	Anger	Impatience Euphoria	Worry	Sadness Grief
Positive Emotion	Courage	Kindness	Love Respect	Calmness Openness	Contentment
Color	Black	Green	Red	Yellow	White
Taste	Salty	Sour	Bitter	Sweet	Spicy/Tart
Smell	Putrid	Rancid	Acrid Burnt	Fragrant	Rotten
Sound	Groaning Sighing	Shouting	Laughing	Singing	Crying
Animal	Bear	Deer	Bird	Monkey	Tiger
Directions	North	East	South	Center	West

Appendix 3: Directions to Face

A wide range of advice is available from both qigong and taiji quan practitioners.

Historically, facing South is the favored position so as to be line with the idea of Emperor's facing to a bright Yang South with his back toward cold Yin North. However, there are still traditional directional options that could be seriously considered when circumstantial inhibitions are not an issue.

EAST

Livia Kohn observes that, in some Daoist practices, "adepts begin with the absorption of qi taken at sunrise in a special chamber set for practice as wells as "burn incense and face east and strike the lithophone nine times to announce the intention of practice" (2008. 158)

In a similar manner, during a 1996 conference on taiji and qigong, attended by one of the authors at the Atomium in Brussels, a Daoist master advised that one "should face east at sunrise to drink the blood of the young sun when it is rising. The *Yijing* also states that "all things issue forth in Chen, which is east" (Chang 1970, 140-41).

WEST

Master Wen-Shan Huang in his classic publication on taiji quan suggests: "Commencing the movements from the north end, first perform the preparatory style by facing west" (1973, 276).

NORTH

Master Jou advises, "Before starting taiji quan, face north" (1980, 112).

NORTH-SOUTH

Giovanni Maciocia cites Marcel Granet (1967) and notes:

> The emperor thus opened himself to receive the influence of heaven, yang, and south. South is therefore like heaven at the top; north is therefore like earth, at the bottom. . . By facing south, the emperor identifies his left with east and his right with west. (1989, 5)

Ken Cohen writes:

> Even the direction you face can influence the efficacy of qigong techniques. A popular traditional practice is for men to always face north, women to face south when practicing qigong. North is the direction of cold, yin. When men face north, they absorb yin-*qi*, balancing their yang. South is the direction of warmth, yang. When women face south, they absorb yang qi, balancing their yin. However, even these rules must occasionally be varied according to circumstances. (1987, 83-84)

He then goes on to say that direction, season and organ can be coordinated and provides a table of five directions.

ANY DIRECTION EXCEPT NORTH

Referring to the *Daoyin jing*, Catherine Despeux writes:

> When one performs the [*daoyin*] exercises for the purpose of therapy, the specific direction toward which they are aimed does not seem to matter. But when they are used as longevity techniques, there are some instructions that detail the geographical orientation for longevity exercises. A smaller number of exercises should be performed facing the direction that corresponds to whatever the season is. Certain directions such as the north should always be avoided, because they evoke the displeasure of the gods. (1989, 251)

Bibliography

Beinfeld, Harriet, and Efrem Korngold. 1991. *Between Heaven and Earth: A Guide to Chinese Medicine*. New York: Ballantine Books.

Bin, Hu. 1982. *A Brief Introduction to the Science of Breathing Exercise*. Hong Kong: Hai Feng Publishing Company.

Cen, Yuefang. 1996. *Chinese Qigong Essentials*. Beijing: New World Press.

Chang, Chung-yuan. 2011. *Creativity and Taoism: A Study of Chinese Philosophy, Art and Poetry*. London: Singing Dragon

Chang, Dr. Stephen T. 1986. *The Complete System of Self-Healing Internal Exercises*. San Francisco: Tao Publishing.

Cheng, Francois. 1994. *Empty and Full the Language of Chinese Painting*. Boston: Shambala Press.

Chia, Mantak, and Maneewan Chia. 2007. *Fusion of the Five Elements: Meditations for Transforming Negative Emotions*. Rochester, Vt.: Destiny Books.

Cleary, Thomas. 1993. *The Essential Tao: An Initiation into the Heart of Taoism through the Authentic Tao Te Ching and the Inner Teachings of Chuang Tzu*. New York: Harper Collins.

Cohen, Kenneth S. 1997. *The Way of Qigong: The Art and Science of Chinese Energy Healing*. New York: Ballantine Books.

Despeux, Catherine. 1979. *Zhao Bizhen: Traité d'alchimie et de physiologie taoïste*. Paris: Guy Trédaniel.

———. 1989. "Gymnastics: The Ancient Tradition." In *Daoist Meditation and Longevity Techniques*, edited by Livia Kohn, 225-61. Ann Arbor: University of Michigan, Center for Chinese Studies.

———. 2004. "La gymnastique *daoyin* dans la Chine ancienne." *Études chinoises* 23: 45-86.

Dhiegh, Khigh Alx. 1973. *The Eleventh Wing: An Exposition of the Dynamics of I Ching for Now*. New York: Dell Publishing.

Ebrey, Patricia Buckley, ed. 1993. *Chinese Civilization A Sourcebook*. New York: The Free Press.

Eliade, Mircea. 2004. *Shamanism: Archaic Techniques of Ecstasy*. Princeton: Princeton University Press.

Goldschmidt, Walter. 1960. *Exploring the Ways of Mankind*. New York: Holt Rinehart and Winston.

Granet, Marcel. 1967. *La pensée chinoise*. Paris: Albin Michael.

Harper, Donald. 2009. *Early Chinese Medical Literature: The Mawangdui Medical Manuscripts*. London: Routledge.

Hicks, Angela, John Hicks, and Peter Mole. 2007. *Five Element Constitutional Acupuncture*. London: Churchill Livingstone.

Huang, Alfred. 1998. *The Complete I Ching*, Rochester, Vt: Inner Traditions.

Huang, Wen-Shan. 1973. *Fundamentals of Tai Chi Chuan*. Hong Kong: Sky Book Company.

Johnson, Jerry Alan. 2005. *Chinese Medical Qi Gong Therapy: Energetic Anatomy and Physiology, Vol 1*. Pacific Grove: International Institute of Medical Qigong.

Jou, Tsung Hwa. 2001. *The Tao of Tai-Chi Chuan: Way to Rejuvenation*. Taipei: Tai Chi Foundation.

Kaptchuk, Ted J. 2000. *The Web that Has No Weaver: Understanding Chinese Medicine*. New York: Congdon & Weed.

Kit, Wong Kiew. 2002. *The Complete Book of Chinese Medicine: A Holistic Approach to Physical, Emotional and Mental Health*. Malaysia: Cosmos.

Kohn, Livia, ed. 1989. *Daoist Meditation and Longevity Techniques*. Ann Arbor: University of Michigan, Center for Chinese Studies.

_____. 2008. *Chinese Healing Exercises: The Tradition of Daoyin*. Honolulu: University of Hawai'i Press.

Master Lam, Kam Chuen. 1991. *The Way of Energy*. New York: Fireside.

Lau, Simon, 1990a, "Basic Guidelines for the Qigong Practitioner." London: Simon Lau Centre.

_____. 1990b, "Martial Arts and Traditional Medicine." London: COMBAT Magazine (December).

Li, Jingwei, and Jianping Zhu. 2010. *An Illustrated Handbook of Chinese Qigong Forms*. Philadelphia: Singing Dragon Press.

Lo, Vivienne. 2007. "Imagining Practice: Sense and Sensuality in Early Chinese Medical Illustration." In *Graphics and Text in the Production of Technical Knowledge in China*, edited by Francisca Bray, Vera Dorofeeva-Lichtmann, and Georges Metailie, 379-423. Leiden: Brill.

_____. 2014. *How to Do the Gibbon Walk: A Translation of the Pulling Book (ca 186 BCE)*. Cambridge: Needham Research Institute.

Lynn, Richard John. 1999. *The Classic of Way and Virtue: A New Translation of the Tao-Te Ching of Laozi as Interpreted by Wang Bi*. New York: Columbia University Press.

Maciocia, Giovanni. 1989. *The Foundations of Chinese Medicine: A Comprehensive Text for Acupuncturists and Herbalists*. New York: Churchill Livingstone.

_____. 2009. *The Psyche in Chinese Medicine: Treatment of Emotional and Mental Disharmonies with Acupuncture and Chinese Herbs*. London: Churchill Livingstone.

Mitchell, Annie, and Maggie Cormack. 1998. *The Therapeutic Relationship in Complementary Medicine*. London: Churchill Livingstone.

Myss, Caroline. 2003. *Sacred Contracts: Awakening Your Divine Potential*. New York: Three Rivers Press.

Ni, Hua-Ching. 2003, *The Complete Works of Lao Tzu*. Los Angeles: Seven Star Communications.

Palmer, David A. 2007. *Qigong Fever: Body, Science and Utopia in China*. New York: Columbia University Press.

Parker, Jerry Alan. 2002. *Chinese Medical Qigong Therapy (Volume 1): Energetic Anatomy and Physiology*. Pacific Grove: International Institute of Medical Qigong.

Pirog, John E. 1996. *The Practical Applications of Meridian Style Acupuncture*. Berkley: Pacific View Press.

Soo, Chee. 1986. *The Taoist Ways of Healing: The Chinese Art of Pa Chin Hsien*. Wellingborough: The Aquarian Press.

Tung, Timothy. 1981. *Wushu! The Chinese Way to Family Health & Fitness*. New York: Simon and Schuster.

Veith, Ilza. 2002. *The Yellow Emperor's Classic of Internal Medicine*. Berkeley: University of California Press.

Wang, Xuanjie, and J. P. C. Moffett. 1994. *Traditional Chinese Therapeutic Exercises – Standing Pole*. Beijing: Foreign Languages Press.

Watts, Alan. 1975. *Tao: The Watercourse Way*. New York: Pantheon Books.

Welch, Holmes. 1957. *Taoism: The Parting of the Way*. Boston: Beacon Press.

Wiseman, Nigel, and Andrew Ellis. 1996. *Fundamentals of Chinese Medicine*. Brookline Massachusetts: Paradigm Publications.

Wong, Eva. 1997. *Taoism: A Complete Introduction*. Boston: Shambhala.

Wu, Zong, and Mao Li. 1992. *Ancient Way to Keep Fit*. Bolinas, Calif.: Shelter Publications.

Yang, Dolly. 2018. "Prescribing 'Guiding and Pulling': The Institutionalization of Therapeutic Exercise in Sui China (581-618 CE)." Ph. D. Diss., University College, London.

Yu, Gongbao. 1995. *Chinese Qigong Illustrated*. Beijing: New World Press.

The Authors

Ronald (Ron) Smith holds degrees from from Princeton University and the University of Southern California. During his military tenure, he was a Senior Fellow at Harvard's John F. Kennedy School of Government. Ron served twenty-nine years in the United States Air Force, nearly half of that time living abroad. Retiring as a colonel in 1998, he remained in Belgium to take a management position in the North Atlantic Treaty Organization.

In a life-changing event, one of his daughter's teachers in Belgium, co-author Tony Carmone, introduced Ron's family to Master Li Changduo and Madam Hu Yang. Master Li studied at Shenyang Sports University, was a member of the Beijing Wushu Team and won two national championships in 1980 and 1981 competing with the Ji (Chinese Halberd). Sadly, he passed away on September 11 2012. His wife, Hu Yang, a particularly creative, but private person, was university trained and also received instruction from Master Li.

For the next eight years, Ron studied Yang-style taiji quan and qigong with them three times a week. Over time, Madam Hu taught other forms such as Eight Pieces of Brocade, Five Animals' Frolics, *Yijin jing*, and *daoyin* movements, specifically those based on the forty-four depictions in the Mawangdui tapestry from the Han Dynasty, which is the main subject of this book.

Eventually, Master Li and Madam Hu asked Ron to teach their classes when they travelled to China or around Europe. Later, Tony and Ron team-taught taiji quan and energy work to expatriates in Belgium. In 2006, Ron and his wife moved to North Texas where they practiced massage therapy for a number of years. In tandem, Ron taught thousands of taiji quan classes at senior centers, the YMCA, assisted care facilities, and in parks. Far from his original teachers, he sought further instruction from books, videos and occasional weekend classes with available teachers. In the end, he recalled the sage advice from his teachers in Belgium: your master is within you now.

Antonio (Tony) Carmone received his BA in Education and Master's Degree in English from Providence College. He earned his Doctorate from the University of Santo Tomas, Manila, Philippines, upon competition of his dissertation on the Confucian, Daoist, and Legalist influences upon the Chinese classical novel, *The Romance of the Three Kingdoms*.

Tony started his lifelong dedication to the martial arts by joining the Uechi-ryu Karate Association (Matson Academy) with Sensei Charles Earle as his instructor in 1964. He was promoted to Shodan.

Tony had the opportunity to learn from respected martial arts masters during a long career as teacher and administrator with the Department of Overseas School System in the Philippines, Taiwan, Korea, Brussels, and London. He had the honor to be taught the Praying Mantis by Master Su Yu-chang in Taiwan, the excitement of practicing Arnis with Master Orlando Centeno in the Philippines, and Tibetan White Crane with Dr. Ismael Lee Chuy and Mr. Eduardo Co, of the Pak Hok Ngai Yuk Tong Chinese Martial Arts Institute. Then, in 1990, he had the privilege of studying *Wing Chun* and qigong under the instruction of Master Simon Lau at Eastern Horizons Studios in London.

The assignment to Brussels served to expand Tony's knowledge of taiji quan. After receiving instruction from Master Li Changduo, Madame Hu Yang, Master Kai-Han Lo, and Madame Gei-Lin Liu, Tony and Ron taught Taijiquan classes together in Brussels.

After his retirement from the Department of Defense Overseas Schools, Tony sought more insight into the underpinnings of *qigong*, *Taijiquan* and Shaolin. He attended the London College of Traditional Acupuncture and Oriental Medicine, receiving a Licentiate Diploma in *Tuina*, and subsequently received a Bachelor of Science in Acupuncture at the University of Portsmouth.

Tony is more recently studying Wu-style taiji quan and qigong with Master Leng Tang in Bradenton, Florida, as well as being instructed by Master Freddie Van Hove from Brussels, Belgium. Tony and Ron have been training and collaborating together since they first met in the late 1990s. For both, learning and cherishing the Art is a never-ending fascination.

Index

Acupuncture points: *baihui* (Hundred Meeting), 60, 70; *laogong* (labor palace), 60, 70, 88, 114; *mingmen* (Gate of Life), 36, 74; *yongquan* (Bubbling Spring), 50, 56, 90, 112; *yunmen* (Cloud Gate), 34; *zhongfu* (Middle Manson), 34

animal movements: Bear Drops, 66, 128; Bear Ramble/Amble, 10, 112, 123; Bird Stretch, 92; Chicken Stretch, 92; Crane Call, 3, 10, 72, 78, 130; Dragon Ascending, 3, 82, 130; Gibbon Jump/Shouting, 3, 110; Merlin, 118, 139; Monkey Bawling, 3, 97, 100, 128; Praying Mantis, 40, 128, 129; Tiger Backs into Cave, 84; Turtle Move, 114, 126, 130

atomium, 149

bells, 138

breathing: 7, 8, 12, 14, 17-20, 49, 56, 64, 76, 122, 124-25, 130, 136, 140-41; abdominal, 8, 18-20; Boulder, 140-41; fetal, 18-19; reverse abdominal, 8, 18-20; unconscious, 18

Chang, Stephen, 147

Chang Tsao, 121

Changsha, 4-5

Chinese Methuselah, 11

chui (healing sound), 20

cinnabar/elixir field, 14

cleansing: 92, 94, 106, 140; breath, 136; ritual, 137

Confucius, 12

Dai, Marquis of, 4

dantian, 14

Diagram of Guiding and Pulling, 5; reconstruction of, 7

Daodejing, 12, 124

Daoism, 1, 11-12, 15, 137

Daoyin, history of, 1-2. 5, 9, 11; 15; as possible supplement 135; ritual preparation for, 137, 139-140; incantation of, 144; direction to face while doing, 147, 150

de (virtue), 16, 138

Despeux, Catherine, 9, 11, 150

divine connections, 138-39

dragon, 3, 9, 82, 78, 130, 139

Eight Pieces of Brocade, 9, 147

elixir field: 14; pulling and guiding into, 21; smiling into, 22. 128; in movement instructions, 27, 32, 34, 36, 38, 40, 42, 44, 46, 50, 56, 58, 60, 63-64, 66, 68, 70, 74, 76, 80, 84, 88, 90, 92, 94, 98, 104-106, 108, 110, 112, 114, 127, 128

emotions, 13-14, 21, 22, 100, 102, 128, 133, 141, 145

emperor, 11-12, 124, 138, 150

156 / Index

essence (*jing*), 14-15, 20-21; affected by *shen*, 15; fresh, 21, 26-28, 30, 32, 34, 36, 38, 40, 42, 44-45, 46, 52, 60, 67-68, 70, 78, 88, 90, 94, 104, 112, 123, 127; stale, 21, 25, 47, 73, 94, 127

fang literature, 5, 12

Five Animals' Frolics, 2, 9, 12, 146

five phases (*wuxing*) 13-14, 66, 139, 148

Forty-Nine Prescriptions of the Ming, 10

guiding and pulling: 5-6, 21, 42, 48, 94, 102, 127, 134; energetic process, 21

Han dynasty, 4-5, 146

Harper, Donald, 5, 8, 10-13, 20, 23, 117-18, 142

healing sounds: 20, 28, 56, 64; *chui* (chway), 20, 56, 85; *hu* (hoo), 20, 28, 56, 66, 85, 94, 100, 110; *xu* (shoe), 20, 28, 56, 66, 70-71, 85, 94, 100, 102

heart-mind, 1-20, 114

hu (healing sound), 20, 28

Hu Bin, 18

Hu Yang, 10, 25

Ni, Hua-Ching, 124

Hua Tuo, 9, 12, 142

Huangdi neijing suwen (The Yellow Emperor's Inner Classic), 11, 12, 124

incense, 144, 149

Jiangling, Zhangjianshan, 5

jing, see essence

Jou, Tsung-Hwa, 23, 136

Khigh, Alx, Dhiegh, 139

Kohn, Livia, 4-5, 10-11, 126, 137, 149

Li, Chancellor, 4

lithophone, 149

Luo, Hongxian, 147

Maciocia, Giovanni, 14-15, 22, 138, 149

magic, 5, 16, 118, 135

Mawangdui, 4-6, 9, 11-13, 122, 139

Master Redpine, 11

medical qigong, 13

medical texts, 5, 7

Merlin, 118, 139

Ming dynasty, 12, 147

Mitchell, Annie, and McCormack, Maggie, 131

monkey, 3, 9, 110, 139; Bawling, 3, 97, 100, 128

Myss, Caroline, 131

Ningfengzi, 11

numbering system, 10

Pace of Yu, 121-23, 129

Pengzu, 11

Praying Mantis, 40, 128-29

pu (uncarved block), 15

Pulling the Eight Radial Cords, 104

qi: 1, 4-5, 7, 11, 14-15, 17, 19-21, 26, 28, 54, 56, 58, 60-61, 68, 70, 76, 84, 88-89, 97-98, 104, 114, 116, 121, 126, 130, 136, 145, 149-50; flow of, 21, 84; as post-heaven essence, 14; as vapor, 6, 7, 11, 121

qigong, 1, 11-13, 17, 19, 146, 149-50

Qianjin yaofan, (Essential Prescriptions for Emergencies Worth a Thousand Pieces of Gold), 9, 146

Quegu shiqi (Abstaining from Grain and Ingesting *Qi*), 7, 20

ritual, 2, 122, 132, 137-38

self-care: 22, 131-33; contract, 131-33, 142; plan, 2, 132

shaman(s): 9, 11, 22-23, 132, 135; dance of, 128; form of, 128-129; as healers, 128; journey of, 135; as physicians, 121-22

Shang dynasty, 126

shen (spirit), 14-15, 20, 124, 146

Shen Shou, 146

Shizi, 122

sounds, *see* healing sounds

Southern Song dynasty, 9, 147

Spiritual-Emotional, 21, 26

standing pole (like a tree), 124

su (simplicity), 16

Sun Simiao, 22, 146

Sui dynasty, 12

Swirling *Qi*, 38

taiji quan, 1, 17, 149

Tang Dynasty, 146

Taiqing Daoyin yangsheng jing (Great Clarity Scripture of Healing Exercists and Nourishing Life), 12

three treasures (*sanbao*), 14, 20, 132

tiger, 9, 84, 139, 148

Traditional Chinese Medicine, 11, 13-14, 131

triple heater (burner, warmer) (*sanjiao*), 14, 56

tu (chart), 1, 5

uncarved block, 3, 15, 121, 128, 135, 144-45

vapor, 6-7, 11, 121

virtue, 15-16, 142

Vivienne Lo, 5, 8, 10, 146

Wang Ziqiao, 11

Watts, Alan, 15-16

Welch, Holmes, 15

wuqinxi (Five Animals' Frolics), 2, 9, 12, 146

wuji, 23, 125

wuwei, 15

xian (immortal, transcendent), 11

Xin Zhui, 4

xu (healing sound), 20

Yang style, 116

Yangsheng fang Daoyin fa (The *Yangsheng* Recipes: The *Daoyin* Methods), 12

Yijing (Book of Changes), 4, 12, 149

Yinshu (Pulling Book), 5, 8- 9, 12, 20, 146

yin and yang, 1, 3, 8, 13, 15, 44, 88, 124, 138

Yinyang shiyi mai jiujing yiben (Cauterization Canon of the

Eleven Yin and Yang Vessels, 8

zhanzhuang (standing posture), 124-26

Zhao Bichen, 15

Zhouli (Rites of Zhou), 9

Zhubing yuanhou lun (Treatise on the Origins and Symptoms of Medical Disorders), 12-13

www.ingramcontent.com/pod-product-compliance
Lightning Source LLC
Chambersburg PA
CBHW032027230426
43671CB00005B/222